Vitamin D

Vin Tangpricha
Editor

Vitamin D

A Clinical Casebook

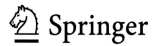 Springer

Editor
Vin Tangpricha
Emory University
Atlanta, GA, USA

ISBN 978-3-319-26174-4   ISBN 978-3-319-26176-8   (eBook)
DOI 10.1007/978-3-319-26176-8

Library of Congress Control Number: 2015960955

Springer Cham Heidelberg New York Dordrecht London

Springer International Publishing AG Switzerland is part of Springer
Science+Business Media (www.springer.com)

Preface

Interest in vitamin D has dramatically increased over the past several decades. From the beginning, vitamin D was incorrectly named a vitamin when later it was discovered to be a member of the steroid hormone family. Over time, the vitamin D receptor was discovered along its major circulating form, 25-hydroxyvitamin D, and its hormonal ligand, 1,25-dihydroxyvitamin D. Classically, vitamin D was known to be important for enhancing intestinal absorption of calcium; however, interest grew in vitamin D when it was determined that vitamin D may be utilized by other tissues of the body. The role of vitamin D in cancer, cardiovascular disease, infection, and other conditions is still under investigation.

Physicians and health-care providers encounter patients with a variety of diseases that require different forms of vitamin D. There are a variety of formations of vitamin D that may have an important role in clinical practice today. The purpose of this case book is to present a practicing physician with a number of different cases commonly seen in practice that require different forms of vitamin D therapy. This book presents in a case-based format several cases ranging from simple vitamin D deficiency to patients with genetic diseases that disrupt vitamin D metabolism. These case presentations should help the reader comprehend the importance of vitamin D in human health.

Atlanta, GA, USA   Vin Tangpricha

Contents

Contributors

Suephy C. Chen, MD, MS Emory University Department of Dermatology, Atlanta, GA, USA

Supavit Chesdachai, MD Mahidol University, Bangkok, Thailand

Tina Constantin, MD Emory University School of Medicine, Atlanta, GA, USA

Malcolm D. Kearns, MD University of Pennsylvania, Philadelphia, PA, USA

Maria Lee, MD Emory University School of Medicine, Atlanta, GA, USA

Kevin Man Hin Luk Emory University School of Medicine, Atlanta, GA, USA

Oranan Siwamogsatham, MD Samitivej Children's Hospital, Bangkok Hospital Group, Bangkok, Thailand

Vin Tangpricha, MD, PhD Emory University School of Medicine, Atlanta, GA, USA

Chapter 1
Young Woman with Vitamin D Deficiency

Supavit Chesdachai and Vin Tangpricha

Case Presentation

A 30-year-old Caucasian woman presented to the rheumatology clinic regarding her diffuse joint and muscle pain for 6 months. She described her pain as confined to her lower back and both lower extremities. The pain progressed in the last 6 weeks to the point that she felt aches all over her body especially in her joints during her daily activity. She also reported malaise, burning sensation in both arms, and muscle weakness in the proximal limbs. The pain impacted her lifestyle and daily activities, limited her ambulation, and resulted in weight gain due to lack of exercise. She denied history of morning stiffness, joint swelling, rash, or photosensitivity.

S. Chesdachai, M.D. (✉)
Mahidol University, Bangkok, Thailand
e-mail: s.chesdachai@gmail.com

V. Tangpricha, M.D., Ph.D.
Emory University School of Medicine, Atlanta, GA, USA
e-mail: vin.tangpricha@emory.edu

© Springer International Publishing Switzerland 2016
V. Tangpricha (ed.), *Vitamin D*,
DOI 10.1007/978-3-319-26176-8_1

1

She had a history of depression, anxiety, and eating disorder for which she takes desvenlafaxine (Pristiq®) 100 mg per day. Her past medical history was also significant for a kidney stone in the past 10 years and traumatic fractures on several occasions in her wrist, thumb, and foot associated with sport activities 10 years ago. She once was diagnosed with Lyme's disease two decades ago and was given tetracycline with full recovery of her symptoms. Her family members were all in good state of health except for high blood pressure in her parents.

She was a well-appearing Caucasian woman. Her physical examination revealed mild pretibial tenderness, no joint swelling. Her vertebral bones were not tender to palpitation. The alignment and range of motion of her joints were normal. Her body mass index (BMI) was 30.5 kg/m². Examinations of other systems were within normal limits.

Her laboratory findings were within the normal ranges except her total serum 25-hydroxyvitamin D (25(OH)D) level was 6.8 ng/mL. Her parathyroid hormone level (PTH) was 28 pg/mL, which was within the normal range. Her antinuclear antibody (ANA), anti-double-stranded DNA antibody (anti-dsDNA), and rheumatoid factor (RF) were negative. Her X-rays of hands and feet were normal. Her bone mineral density (BMD) was within the reference range for young women at the hip and spine.

Her additional history related to her vitamin D status was that she reported no issues with her digestive system. She spends approximately half an hour per week in direct sunlight without wearing any sunscreen and she does not take any additional supplements or vitamin D-containing food. Given the extremely low serum 25(OH)D concentration, she was referred to an endocrinologist for further evaluation and treatment.

Diagnosis and Assessment

This patient presented with signs and symptoms compatible with vitamin D deficiency and osteomalacia. Her low serum 25(OH)D was diagnostic of a severe vitamin D deficiency. There are several etiologies for vitamin D deficiency in a young adult. Malabsorption from bariatric surgery or from other bowel surgery can result in vitamin D deficiency. Other intestinal diseases that can result in malabsorption of vitamin D include celiac sprue and cystic fibrosis. Insufficient dietary consumption of vitamin D-containing foods and inadequate sunlight exposure are also very common among children and adults as very few foods contain vitamin D naturally. Furthermore, a modern lifestyle associated with limited outdoor activity can also reduce the cutaneously produced vitamin D in the skin. Medications such as anticonvulsants, for example, phenytoin, can cause vitamin D deficiency by increasing the catabolism of vitamin D [1]. In our case presentation, the etiology for the severe vitamin D deficiency was a combination of lack of dietary intake and inadequate sun light exposure.

Management

Vitamin D deficiency should be treated with oral vitamin D supplements. According to the Endocrine Society's 2011 Clinical Practice Guidelines on Vitamin D [2], one approach to correct vitamin D deficiency is by prescribing ergocalciferol or cholecalciferol 50,000 IU (1.25 mg) oral capsule once or twice a week for 8 weeks. A repeat serum 25(OH)D concentration after 8 weeks of treatment should be checked to confirm a good response.

In order to maintain adequate vitamin D status, the patient should adjust her lifestyle to increase outdoor activity to include sensible sunlight exposure and to increase intake of vitamin D-containing foods. The Endocrine Society recommends 1500–2000 IU of vitamin D as a supplement if dietary intake is inadequate.

Outcome

After 2 months of vitamin D treatment, her symptoms improved. She still has some minimal lower extremity discomfort but she can perform her daily life activities without excessive muscle pain or weakness. Her total serum 25(OH)D concentration reached 30 ng/mL at the end of week 8. She is followed every 6 months in clinic to ensure adequate vitamin D status.

Discussion and Literature Review

Vitamin D deficiency impacts more than one billion people around the world [3]. Two important sources of vitamin D are from adequate dietary intake and cutaneous production of vitamin D in the skin. Exposure to sunlight is the major source of vitamin D for most humans, as very few foods contain vitamin D. Individuals living near the equator still have high prevalence of vitamin D deficiency likely due to increased indoor activities associated with a modern lifestyle [3–5]. Vitamin D synthesis is initiated by exposure of 7-dehydrocholesterol (7-DHC) to UVB (wavelength, 290–315 nm) which is then converted to previtamin D and then vitamin D_3 via a thermally induced reaction in the skin [6]. Vitamin D_3 either from diet or skin then binds to the vitamin D-binding protein in the blood and hydroxylated via hepatic cytochrome P450 vitamin D 25-hydroxylase (25-OHase or CYP27A1) in the liver to become 25-hydroxyvitamin D (25(OH)D). The next step of hydroxylation occurs in proximal tubule of the kidney via renal cytochrome P450 D-1-α-hydroxylase (1-OHase or CYP27B1) to form 1,25-dihydroxyvitamin D ($1,25(OH)_2D$) which is the active form of vitamin D [7].

Vitamin D has an important role in both skeletal and extraskeletal health. It plays a role in the intestinal absorption of calcium and phosphorus. Low levels of vitamin D will result in elevations of parathyroid hormone which increases the resorption of bone leading to decreased mineralization and increased risk of osteomalacia, osteoporosis, and bone fractures [8]. Vitamin D also has a major role in many extraskeletal conditions such as cancer, infection, autoimmune disease, diabetes, and cardiovascular disease [9, 10].

The clinical manifestations of vitamin D deficiency in adults include muscle aches, pain, and proximal muscle weakness [11–13]. These symptoms are usually misdiagnosed as fibromyalgia. Bone pain and increased risk of bone fracture are the manifestations of osteomalacia stemming from vitamin D deficiency. The physical examination is usually unspecific except pain at either the spine or sternum upon pressure. Patients who present with nonspecific muscle pain should be evaluated for vitamin D deficiency.

The best way to evaluate vitamin D status is measurement of a serum 25(OH)D concentration. A serum 25(OH)D concentration of less than 20 ng/mL (50 nmol/L) represents vitamin D deficiency. Serum 25(OH)D concentrations between 21 and 29 ng/mL (52–72 nmol/L) are considered vitamin D insufficient. Serum 25(OH)D above 30 ng/mL (75 nmol/L) is desired. Vitamin D deficiency/insufficiency is often associated with elevations in parathyroid hormone concentrations, termed secondary hyperparathyroidism [1, 14, 15].

According to the 2011 Endocrine Society Guidelines, screening for vitamin D deficiency should be performed in patients at risk for vitamin D deficiency such as patients with malabsorption, osteoporosis, or obesity [2]. Patients with vitamin D deficiency should be treated with 50,000 IU vitamin D_2 or D_3 once a week or 6000 IU vitamin D_2 or D_3 once per day for 8 weeks followed by maintenance therapy of vitamin D 1500–2000 IU/day to maintain a serum 25(OH)D concentration above 30 ng/mL [2, 16].

Sunlight exposure is an important determinant of vitamin D status. The factors that contribute to vitamin D product are skin pigmentation, season, sunscreen, and latitude. Sensible sun exposure 5–30 min, 2 times per week in between 10 a.m. and 3 p.m., is considered as adequate [1, 4]. Vitamin D from diet is usually not enough to satisfy the daily requirement of vitamin D. Foods that naturally contain vitamin D include oily fish, mushrooms, and egg yolks. Fortified food may contain either ergocalciferol or cholecalciferol but in limited amounts, typically 100 IU of vitamin D per serving [17–19].

Clinical Pearls and Pitfalls

- Vitamin D deficiency is very common among the population even in young healthy individuals.
- A serum 25-hydroxyvitamin D (25(OH)D) is the best marker to assess vitamin D status. A serum 25(OH)D of less than 20 ng/mL is considered as vitamin D deficiency. A serum 25(OH)D in the range of 21–29 ng/mL is considered vitamin D insufficient and more than 30 ng/mL is considered vitamin D sufficient.

- Clinical manifestations of vitamin D deficiency are subtle. In adults, the symptoms that suggest vitamin D deficiency are muscle and bone pain as well as generalized muscle weakness.
- Treatment of vitamin D deficiency can be accomplished with higher dose vitamin D supplements followed by maintenance of vitamin D to prevent vitamin D deficiency.

Suggested Reading

1. Holick MF. Vitamin D deficiency. N Engl J Med. 2007;357 (3):266–81.
2. Holick MF, Binkley NC, Bischoff-Ferrari HA, Gordon CM, Hanley DA, Heaney RP, et al. Evaluation, treatment, and prevention of vitamin D deficiency: an endocrine society clinical practice guideline. J Clin Endocrinol Metab. 2011;96(7): 1911–30.
3. Hossein-Nezhad A, Holick MF. Vitamin D for health: a global perspective. Mayo Clin Proc. 2013;88(7):720–55.

References

1. Holick MF. Vitamin D deficiency. N Engl J Med. 2007;357(3): 266–81.
2. Holick MF, Binkley NC, Bischoff-Ferrari HA, Gordon CM, Hanley DA, Heaney RP, et al. Evaluation, treatment, and prevention of vitamin D deficiency: an endocrine society clinical practice guideline. J Clin Endocrinol Metab. 2011;96(7):1911–30.
3. Palacios C, Gonzalez L. Is vitamin D deficiency a major global public health problem? J Steroid Biochem Mol Biol. 2014;144(Pt A):138–45.
4. Nimitphong H, Holick MF. Vitamin D status and sun exposure in southeast Asia. Dermatoendocrinology. 2013;5(1):34–7.
5. Siwamogsatham O, Ongphiphadhanakul B, Tangpricha V. Vitamin D deficiency in Thailand. J Clin Transl Endocrinol. 2015;2(1):48–9.
6. Wacker M, Holick MF. Sunlight and vitamin D: a global perspective for health. Dermatoendocrinology. 2013;5(1):51–108.
7. Christakos S, Ajibade DV, Dhawan P, Fechner AJ, Mady LJ. Vitamin D: metabolism. Endocrinol Metab Clin North Am. 2010;39(2):243–53. table of contents.

8. Grober U, Spitz J, Reichrath J, Kisters K, Holick MF. Vitamin D: update 2013: From rickets prophylaxis to general preventive healthcare. Dermatoendocrinology. 2013;5(3):331–47.

9. Wacker M, Holick MF. Vitamin D – effects on skeletal and extraskeletal health and the need for supplementation. Nutrients. 2013;5(1):111–48.

10. Holick MF. Vitamin D: extraskeletal health. Endocrinol Metab Clin North Am. 2010;39(2):381–400. table of contents.

11. Holick MF. Vitamin D, deficiency: what a pain it is. Mayo Clin Proc. 2003;78(12):1457–9.

12. Plotnikoff GA, Quigley JM. Prevalence of severe hypovitaminosis D in patients with persistent, nonspecific musculoskeletal pain. Mayo Clin Proc. 2003;78(12):1463–70.

13. Heidari B, Shirvani JS, Firouzjahi A, Heidari P, Hajian-Tilaki KO. Association between nonspecific skeletal pain and vitamin D deficiency. Int J Rheum Dis. 2010;13(4):340–6.

14. Chapuy MC, Preziosi P, Maamer M, Arnaud S, Galan P, Hercberg S, et al. Prevalence of vitamin D insufficiency in an adult normal population. Osteoporos Int. 1997;7(5):439–43.

15. Jorde R, Grimnes G. Vitamin D and health: the need for more randomized controlled trials. The Journal of steroid biochemistry and molecular biology. 2015;148:269–74.

16. Holick MF, Chen TC. Vitamin D deficiency: a worldwide problem with health consequences. Am J Clin Nutr. 2008;87(4):1080s–6.

17. Hossein-nezhad A, Holick MF. Vitamin D for health: a global perspective. Mayo Clin Proc. 2013;88(7):720–55.

18. Tangpricha V. Vitamin D in food and supplements. Am J Clin Nutr. 2012;95(6):1299–300.

19. Cashman KD. Vitamin D: dietary requirements and food fortification as a means of helping achieve. J Steroid Biochem Mol Biol. 2015;148:19–26.

Chapter 2
Vitamin D Deficiency in Infants

Oranan Siwamogsatham and Vin Tangpricha

Case Presentation

A 6-month-old male Turkish infant presented with fever and three recent episodes of generalized seizures, each episode lasting for approximately 5 min. This patient was reported well until the day of admission when his skin felt warm followed by an episode of generalized seizures. He was born full term and was exclusively breastfed since birth, with no vitamin supplementation. Family history was negative for epilepsy. His parents were not

O. Siwamogsatham, M.D. (✉)
Samitivej Children's Hospital, Bangkok Hospital Group,
488 Srinakarin Road, Suanluang, Bangkok 10250, Thailand
e-mail: oranan.w@gmail.com

V. Tangpricha, M.D., Ph.D.
Emory University School of Medicine, Atlanta, GA, USA
e-mail: vin.tangpricha@emory.edu

© Springer International Publishing Switzerland 2016   9
V. Tangpricha (ed.), *Vitamin D*,
DOI 10.1007/978-3-319-26176-8_2

cosanguineous. His mother followed the Islamic faith and dressed with most of her skin covered. She did not take vitamin supplements during pregnancy or lactation. On examination, the infant was drowsy after the epileptic spell. The temperature was 38 °C, the blood pressure 90/45 mmHg, the pulse 140 beats per minute, and the respiratory rate 40 breaths per minute. His weight, height, and head circumference were in 97th percentile for age. There was no bulging of the anterior fontanelle. Auscultation of lung sounds revealed coarse crepitation and rhonchi bilaterally. The patient did not have any dysmorphic facial features or skeletal deformities on exam. Neurological examinations were normal.

Diagnosis/Assessment

Complete blood count showed leukocytosis (WBC 36,230 per mm^3; neutrophils 27 %, lymphocytes 58 %, monocytes 13 %). Biochemical studies revealed normal plasma glucose (106 mg/dL), low serum calcium (5.8 mg/dL), normal serum phosphorus (5.2 mg/dL), and magnesium (1.8 mg/dL). Serum parathyroid hormone was elevated (117.7 pg/mL). Serum 25-hydroxyvitamin D (25(OH)D) was undetectable (<3 ng/mL). Serum alkaline phosphatase was normal for age (240 U/L). Serum electrolytes and kidney function were normal. A radiograph of the chest revealed perihilar infiltration. The respiratory panel result was positive for respiratory syncytial virus (RSV). Computer tomography of the brain and the cerebrospinal fluid profiles were normal.

The history of fever-provoked seizure in exclusively breastfed infant coupled with laboratory values that showed hypocalcemia, elevated PTH, and undetectable 25(OH)D level was consistent with the diagnosis of hypocalcemia due to severe vitamin D deficiency. The cause of fever, from the investigations, was consistent with RSV bronchiolitis.

Management/Outcome

Immediate treatment of severe vitamin D deficiency with symptomatic hypocalcemia requires intravenous calcium, oral calcitriol (the hormonal form of vitamin D, 1,25-dihydroxyvitamin D), and oral vitamin D supplementation. In this case, 10 % calcium gluconate 1 mL/kg was promptly given intravenously every 6 h along with oral calcitriol 1 mcg/day, oral calcium containing 500 mg of elemental calcium/day, and oral vitamin D_2 10,000 IU/day. Phenytoin was also administered to control the seizure. Two days after treatment, his serum calcium increased to 7.2 mg/dL. Intravenous calcium was then decreased to 1 mL/kg every 12 h. Four days after treatment, his serum calcium increased into the normal range (8.4 mg/dL). Intravenous calcium was then discontinued and his calcium remained in the normal range (8.8 mg/dL). Oral calcitriol was eventually decreased to a dose of 0.25 mcg/day on day 8 of treatment. His seizure ceased within the first day of starting treatment. He remained on calcitriol 0.25 mcg/day, calcium which contains 500 mg of elemental calcium/day, and vitamin D_2 10,000 IU/day until day 10 of treatment and was then discharged home with oral vitamin D_3 1400 IU/day and 300 mg of elemental calcium/day. Laboratory tests prior to discharge revealed normal calcium (10 mg/dL), normal phosphorus (4.7 mg/dL), and slightly elevated PTH (83.6 pg/mL). After his discharge to home, he went back to his home country and planned a follow-up visit at his home country.

Literature Review

Vitamin D sources in early infancy come from transplacental stores, breast milk, and cutaneous production via sunlight exposure. Maternal vitamin D status is important in determining the vitamin D reserves at birth via placental vitamin D transport and early infancy via breast milk. It is well recognized that maternal vitamin D deficiency during pregnancy and during lactation contributes to the development of vitamin D deficiency and rickets in infancy.

Exclusively breastfed infants of mothers who avoid sunlight and have inadequate vitamin D intake, similar to this case presentation, put their child at risk for developing vitamin D deficiency [1, 2].

The 2010 Institute of Medicine (IOM) recommends a daily vitamin D intake of 400–600 IU/day in pregnant women to achieve the circulating 25(OH)D of 20 ng/mL [3], whereas the Endocrine Society recommends an intake of 1500–2000 IU/day to achieve a circulating 25(OH)D level of more than 30 ng/mL [4]. There are many studies indicate that routine use of prenatal vitamins containing 400 IU of vitamin D does not prevent vitamin D deficiency in pregnant women [5–7]. The Endocrine Society recommends that all pregnant women should take at least a prenatal vitamin containing 400 IU vitamin D per day with a supplement that contains at least 1000 IU vitamin D per day. Studies of vitamin D supplementation in pregnancy showed that at least 1000–2000 IU/day of vitamin D may be needed to ensure serum 25(OH)D above 20 ng/mL [6, 8]. Two recent RCT showed that vitamin D intake of 4000 IU/day during pregnancy was most effective in achieving serum 25(OH)D concentrations of 32 ng/mL or more throughout pregnancy without increase risk of toxicity in pregnant women and their neonates [7, 9].

Post-partum during lactation, the Endocrine Society recommends that women should take at least a multivitamin containing 400 IU vitamin D along with at least 1000 IU vitamin D supplement every day. In women who exclusively breastfeed, at least 4000–6000 IU/day of vitamin D may be necessary to transfer adequate vitamin D into milk to satisfy the infant's vitamin D requirements. Thus, at minimum, lactating women may need to take vitamin D 1400–1500 IU/day, and to satisfy their infant's requirement, and they may need 4000–6000 IU/day if they choose not to give the infant a vitamin D supplement [4]. A RCT study in lactating women reported that daily vitamin D intake at the dose of 2000 and 4000 IU could achieve sufficient circulatory 25(OH)D level (>30 ng/mL) for mothers. However, infants of mothers ingesting 4000 IU/day of vitamin D exhibited higher 25(OH)D concentrations than infants of mothers ingesting 2000 IU/day of vitamin D [10]. A more recent study showed that a maternal intake vitamin D of 6400 IU/day during lactation was safe and significantly elevates circulating 25(OH)D level in both mothers and nursing infants. These results compared favorably with infants receiving 300–400 IU/day of vitamin D [11].

Human breast milk and unfortified cow's milk contain very little vitamin D naturally. The average amount of vitamin D in human milk and colostrums is approximately 15.9 ± 8.6 IU/L [10]. Thus, infants who are fed only human breast milk are prone to developing vitamin D deficiency. The Endocrine Society recommends that infants require at least 400 IU/day of vitamin D to maximize bone health. However, to ensure blood levels of 25(OH)D consistently above 30 mg/dL, infants may require at least 1000 IU/day of vitamin D [4]. The American Academy of Pediatrics (AAP) recommends that all breast-fed infants, infants who receive a mixture of human milk and formula milk, and any infant who receives <1 L or 1 qt of formula per day need vitamin D supplement of 400 IU/day beginning within the first few days of life and continuing throughout childhood to maintain serum 25(OH)D concentration at >20 ng/mL [12].

Despite daily supplementation with 400 IU as recommended by the AAP guidelines, vitamin D deficiency in infancy is still highly prevalent [13]. Some studies suggested that vitamin D supplementation in infants should be increased above the recommended 400 IU/day especially in winter season and in infants who have high risk of vitamin D deficiency such as in infants born to vitamin D-deficient mothers due to low sunlight exposure, low intake of dairy products, and inadequate vitamin D supplementation during pregnancy and lactation [14–16]. A recent RCT showed that vitamin D supplementation up to 1600 IU/day in infants was safe and resulted in serum 25(OH)D concentrations within the normal range and consistently above 32 ng/mL [16].

Clinical Pearls and Pitfalls

- Vitamin D status of infants is dependent on the mother's vitamin D status early in life.
- Exclusively breastfed infants are at risk for developing vitamin D deficiency since very little vitamin D is contained in breast milk, especially if the mother is vitamin D deficient.
- Supplementation of the infant and of the lactating mother are two approaches to improve vitamin D status of children in early infancy.

Suggested Reading

1. Hollis BW, Johnson D, Hulsey TC, Ebeling M, Wagner CL. Vitamin D supplementation during pregnancy: double-blind, randomized clinical trial of safety and effectiveness. J Bone Miner Res. 2011;26(10):2341–57.
2. Wagner CL, Hulsey TC, Fanning D, Ebeling M, Hollis BW. High-dose vitamin D3 supplementation in a cohort of breastfeeding mothers and their infants: a 6-month follow-up pilot study. Breastfeed Med. 2006;1(2):59–70.
3. Hollis BW1, Wagner CL. Vitamin D and pregnancy: skeletal effects, nonskeletal effects, and birth outcomes. Calcif Tissue Int. 2013;92(2):128–39.

References

1. Andiran N, Yordam N, Ozon A. Risk factors for vitamin D deficiency in breast-fed newborns and their mothers. Nutrition. 2002;18(1):47–50.
2. Bowyer L, Catling-Paull C, Diamond T, Homer C, Davis G, Craig ME. Vitamin D, PTH and calcium levels in pregnant women and their neonates. Clin Endocrinol. 2009;70(3):372–7.
3. Food and Nutrition Board. Standing committee on the scientific evaluation of dietary reference intakes for vitamin D and calcium. Washington, DC: National Academy Press; 2010.
4. Holick MF, Binkley NC, Bischoff-Ferrari HA, Gordon CM, Hanley DA, Heaney RP, et al. Evaluation, treatment, and prevention of vitamin D deficiency: an endocrine society clinical practice guideline. J Clin Endocrinol Metab. 2011;96(7):1911–30.
5. Bodnar LM, Simhan HN, Powers RW, Frank MP, Cooperstein E, Roberts JM. High prevalence of vitamin D insufficiency in black and white pregnant women residing in the northern United States and their neonates. J Nutr. 2007;137(2):447–52.
6. Yesiltepe Mutlu G, Ozsu E, Kalaca S, Yuksel A, Pehlevan Y, Cizmecioglu F, et al. Evaluation of vitamin D supplementation doses during pregnancy in a population at high risk for deficiency. Horm Res Paediatr. 2014;81(6):402–8.
7. Dawodu A, Saadi HF, Bekdache G, Javed Y, Altaye M, Hollis BW. Randomized controlled trial (RCT) of vitamin D supplementation in pregnancy in a population with endemic vitamin D deficiency. J Clin Endocrinol Metab. 2013;98(6):2337–46.

8. Grant CC, Stewart AW, Scragg R, Milne T, Rowden J, Ekeroma A, et al. Vitamin D during pregnancy and infancy and infant serum 25-hydroxyvita-min D concentration. Pediatrics. 2014;133(1):e143–53.

9. Hollis BW, Johnson D, Hulsey TC, Ebeling M, Wagner CL. Vitamin D supplementation during pregnancy: double-blind, randomized clinical trial of safety and effectiveness. J Bone Miner Res. 2011;26(10):2341–57.

10. Hollis BW, Wagner CL. Vitamin D requirements during lactation: high-dose maternal supplementation as therapy to prevent hypovitaminosis D for both the mother and the nursing infant. Am J Clin Nutr. 2004;80 Suppl 6:1752S–8.

11. Wagner CL, Hulsey TC, Fanning D, Ebeling M, Hollis BW. High-dose vitamin D3 supplementation in a cohort of breastfeeding mothers and their infants: a 6-month follow-up pilot study. Breastfeed Med. 2006; 1(2):59–70.

12. Wagner CL, Greer FR, American Academy of Pediatrics Section on B, American Academy of Pediatrics Committee on N. Prevention of rickets and vitamin D deficiency in infants, children, and adolescents. Pediatrics. 2008;122(5):1142–52.

13. Vieth Streym S, Kristine Moller U, Rejnmark L, Heickendorff L, Mosekilde L, Vestergaard P. Maternal and infant vitamin D status during the first 9 months of infant life-a cohort study. Eur J Clin Nutr. 2013;67(10):1022–8.

14. Halicioglu O, Sutcuoglu S, Koc F, Yildiz O, Akman SA, Aksit S. Vitamin D status of exclusively breastfed 4-month-old infants supplemented during different seasons. Pediatrics. 2012;130(4):e921–7.

15. Onal H, Adal E, Alpaslan S, Ersen A, Aydin A. Is daily 400 IU of vitamin D supplementation appropriate for every country: a cross-sectional study. Eur J Nutr. 2010;49(7):395–400.

16. Holmlund-Suila E, Viljakainen H, Hytinantti T, Lamberg-Allardt C, Andersson S, Makitie O. High-dose vitamin D intervention in infants—effects on vitamin D status, calcium homeostasis, and bone strength. J Clin Endocrinol Metab. 2012;97(11):4139–47.

Chapter 3
Vitamin D Deficiency in Cystic Fibrosis

Supavit Chesdachai and Vin Tangpricha

Case Presentation

A 24-year-old Caucasian woman with cystic fibrosis (CF) was referred to the endocrinology clinic for evaluation of vitamin D deficiency. Six years prior to this visit, she had been diagnosed with vitamin D deficiency and osteopenia from a different hospital. She received 50,000 IU of ergocalciferol (vitamin D_2) daily, which did not improve her vitamin D status. She was currently taking 50,000 IU ergocalciferol three times a day. Her total serum 25-hydroxyvitamin D (25(OH)D) level was 24 ng/mL. Her bone mineral density (BMD) was lower than the young adult range; with

S. Chesdachai, M.D. (✉)
Mahidol University, Bangkok, Thailand
e-mail: s.chesdachai@gmail.com

V. Tangpricha, M.D., Ph.D.
Emory University School of Medicine, Atlanta, GA, USA
e-mail: vin.tangpricha@emory.edu

© Springer International Publishing Switzerland 2016
V. Tangpricha (ed.), *Vitamin D*,
DOI 10.1007/978-3-319-26176-8_3

17

T-scores at the hip and spine of less than −2.0. She denied any history of vitamin D deficiency-related symptoms such as bone pain, muscle ache, or past history of fracture.

She has a regular follow-up visits at the CF clinic. Her baseline forced expiratory volume in one second (FEV1) was 43 % of the predicted. She had no sputum production and hemoptysis at her baseline. She was performing activities of daily living (ADL) without limitation as well as denied dyspnea on exertion. She had remote history of pulmonary exacerbation that required twice-yearly hospitalization and received antimicrobial therapy from time to time depending on her respiratory status.

She had cystic fibrosis-related diabetes (CFRD) without fasting hyperglycemia that was diagnosed based on a 2-hour oral glucose tolerance test; she rarely required insulin therapy for her blood glucose control and her hemoglobin A1C had been under 6 %. She was taking pancreatic enzyme supplements for exocrine pancreatic insufficiency related to CF. She was spending less than 30 minutes per day outdoors on a daily basis.

Diagnosis and Assessment

This patient has CF with chronic vitamin D deficiency and osteopenia. There are many etiologies that contribute to vitamin D insufficiency and deficiency in the CF population. Malabsorption from the pancreatic exocrine insufficiency is one of the major causes of vitamin D deficiency in patients with CF [1]. Pancreatic exocrine insufficiency results in electrolyte imbalances across the pancreatic duct epithelium and results in the hyperconcentration of pancreatic fluid leading to obstruction of the pancreatic duct and eventual destruction and fibrosis of the pancreas. The pancreatic insufficiency that ensues results in micronutrient malabsorption especially in fat and fat-soluble vitamins including vitamin D [2]. Several studies have reported that it is difficult to restore normal circulating levels of 25(OH)D in patients with CF [3]. Moreover, patients with CF have decreased hepatic hydroxylation activity which is essential for vitamin D metabolism which further results in low circulating concentrations of (25(OH)D) [4, 5]. Other potential reasons for vitamin D deficiency are decreased vitamin D binding protein, lower body fat mass for vitamin D storage, and inadequate sunlight exposure [1, 4, 5].

Our case patient developed vitamin D deficiency due to fat malabsorption from pancreatic exocrine insufficiency and inadequate sunlight exposure. Vitamin D deficiency also likely contributed to this case's osteopenia.

Management

She was prescribed high-dose ergocalciferol for a period of time; however, that was not able to restore her serum 25(OH)D concentration above 30 ng/mL (75 nmol/L). She was then switched to cholecalciferol 50,000 IU daily for 1 month followed by cholecalciferol 50,000 IU three times a week to maintain her vitamin D status. To address her osteopenia, she was instructed to take calcium supplements along with vitamin D and to improve her lifestyle by routine weight-bearing exercise and diet modification to maintain body weight and to spend more time outdoors in the sun.

Outcome

Many studies demonstrated that low dose of daily ergocalciferol failed to raise the vitamin D levels above 30 ng/mL (75 nmol/L) [3, 6]. Even with higher doses of ergocalciferol supplements, the failure rate of treatment of vitamin D deficiency was still high [7]. In this case, after one month of treatment, her vitamin D level has increased above 30 ng/mL (75 nmol/L), but her BMD was still lower than normal. Her vitamin D levels and BMD will be periodically monitored.

Discussion and Literature Review

Cystic fibrosis is a rare lethal autosomal recessive disease that occurs mostly in Caucasians. The disease results from a mutation of cystic fibrosis transmembrane conductance regulator (CFTR) gene, leading to defects of chloride and water transport across the epithelium, causing thickening of mucous membrane, primarily in the respiratory tract and gastrointestinal tract [8]. Consequently, patients with CF suffer from recurrent pulmonary infections, chronic inflammation of the lungs leading to progressive bronchiectasis, inability to clear pathogenic bacterial from the lungs, and pancreatic insufficiency [9].

Vitamin D deficiency is a very common problem among patients with CF. Up to 90 % of CF patients have vitamin D insufficiency or deficiency, as a consequence of pancreatic exocrine insufficiency [1]. Vitamin D plays an important role in both skeletal and nonskeletal-related health in patients with CF. As in the normal population, when vitamin D status is low, there is less efficient absorption of calcium and phosphorus leading to an increase in parathyroid hormone level and bone resorption [10]. Patients with CF have a high prevalence of osteopenia, osteoporosis, and fractures [11]. However, low bone density is not only due to vitamin D deficiency but also related to many factors including malnutrition, chronic inflammation, glucocorticoid use, reduced physical activity, and delayed puberty or early gonadal failure [12].

Several studies have demonstrated that vitamin D may improve recurrence of pulmonary exacerbations, reduce inflammation, and enhance antimicrobial activity of macrophages [13]. In the Third National Health and Nutrition Examination Survey (NHANES III), vitamin D status was positively associated with lung function in healthy adults [14]. Specifically in CF, two retrospective cohort studies demonstrate that higher vitamin D status was associated with lower rate of pulmonary exacerbation and improved lung function [15, 16]. A randomized, double-blinded, placebo-controlled trial demonstrated that high-dose vitamin D lowered hospitalization rates and improved clinical outcomes in patients with CF [17].

Vitamin D's anti-inflammatory and antibacterial properties may help improve lung pathology in CF patients. Vitamin D can upregulate the production of the antimicrobial peptide cathelicidin (hCAP or LL-37) in macrophages [18]. Furthermore, vitamin D can enhance the antimicrobial activity against airway pathogens such as *Pseudomonas aeruginosa* via LL-37 in CF bronchial epithelial cells [19]. Vitamin D also downregulates proinflammatory cytokines in the macrophages [13, 20] which decreases inflammation in CF lungs. The secondary analysis of a randomized, double-blinded, placebo-controlled trial showed that high dose of vitamin D was able to reduce interleukin-6 (IL-6) and tumor necrotic factor α (TNF-α) levels in the CF patients with pulmonary exacerbation [17, 21]. Further study should be conducted to help determine the benefit of vitamin D supplementation in different aspects.

Similarly to the general population, serum 25(OH)D should be used to determine the vitamin D status in CF population. Annual screening of vitamin D deficiency by measurement of a serum 25(OH)D in all patients with CF, especially at the end of the winter season, is also recommended by the CF Foundation [22]. Vitamin D either in daily or weekly doses should be prescribed to all patients with CF with vitamin D deficiency and insufficiency. The dose of vitamin D is based on the age and initial starting concentration of serum 25(OH)D. Most children and adults should initially start on between 400 and 2000 IU of vitamin D daily and the dose should be increased in a stepwise fashion to ensure a target serum 25(OH)D concentration of at least 30 ng/mL [22].

There is limited evidence regarding the use of tanning beds or UV lamp therapy in patients with CF. One case series of five patients with CF reported that after five times a week of UV lamp therapy for 8 weeks improved vitamin D status [23]. In contrast, two interventional studies showed no difference in these therapies [24, 25].

Clinical Pearls and Pitfalls

- Vitamin D deficiency is very common in patients with CF due to pancreatic exocrine insufficiency and other causes. Vitamin D may play a role not only for the skeleton but also other organs

outside the skeleton including the lung and immune system in patients with CF.
- Vitamin D deficiency is one of the major causes that increase the risk of fractures, osteopenia, and osteoporosis in patients with CF.
- Serum 25(OH)D should be screened annually in all patients with CF, especially at the end of the winter season. High-dose cholecalciferol is recommended for the treatment of vitamin D deficiency in CF.

Suggested Reading

1. Tangpricha V, Kelly A, Stephenson A, Maguiness K, Enders J, Robinson KA, et al. An update on the screening, diagnosis, management, and treatment of vitamin D deficiency in individuals with cystic fibrosis: evidence-based recommendations from the cystic fibrosis foundation. J Clin Endocrinol Metab. 2012; 97(4):1082–93.
2. Hall WB, Sparks AA, Aris RM. Vitamin d deficiency in cystic fibrosis. Int J Endocrinol. 2010;2010:218691.

References

1. Hall WB, Sparks AA, Aris RM. Vitamin d deficiency in cystic fibrosis. Int J Endocrinol. 2010;2010:218691.
2. Couper RT, Corey M, Moore DJ, Fisher LJ, Forstner GG, Durie PR. Decline of exocrine pancreatic function in cystic fibrosis patients with pancreatic sufficiency. Pediatr Res. 1992;32(2):179–82.
3. Rovner AJ, Stallings VA, Schall JI, Leonard MB, Zemel BS. Vitamin D insufficiency in children, adolescents, and young adults with cystic fibrosis despite routine oral supplementation. Am J Clin Nutr. 2007;86(6):1694–9.
4. Mailhot G. Vitamin D, bioavailability in cystic fibrosis: a cause for concern? Nutr Rev. 2012;70(5):280–93.
5. Siwamogsatham O, Alvarez JA, Tangpricha V. Diagnosis and treatment of endocrine comorbidities in patients with cystic fibrosis. Curr Opin Endocrinol Diabetes Obes. 2014;21(5):422–9.

6. Green D, Carson K, Leonard A, Davis JE, Rosenstein B, Zeitlin P, et al. Current treatment recommendations for correcting vitamin D deficiency in pediatric patients with cystic fibrosis are inadequate. J Pediatr. 2008;153(4):554–9.
7. Boyle MP, Noschese ML, Watts SL, Davis ME, Stenner SE, Lechtzin N. Failure of high-dose ergocalciferol to correct vitamin D deficiency in adults with cystic fibrosis. Am J Respir Crit Care Med. 2005;172(2):212–7.
8. Collawn JF, Matalon S. CFTR and lung homeostasis. Am J Physiol Lung Cell Mol Physiol. 2014;307(12):L917–23.
9. Stoltz DA, Meyerholz DK, Welsh MJ. Origins of cystic fibrosis lung disease. N Engl J Med. 2015;372(4):351–62.
10. Holick MF. Vitamin D, deficiency. N Engl J Med. 2007;357 (3):266–81.
11. Paccou J, Zeboulon N, Combescure C, Gossec L, Cortet B. The prevalence of osteoporosis, osteopenia, and fractures among adults with cystic fibrosis: a systematic literature review with meta-analysis. Calcif Tissue Int. 2010;86(1):1–7.
12. Aris RM, Merkel PA, Bachrach LK, Borowitz DS, Boyle MP, Elkin SL, et al. Guide to bone health and disease in cystic fibrosis. J Clin Endocrinol Metab. 2005;90(3):1888–96.
13. Herscovitch K, Dauletbaev N, Lands LC. Vitamin D as an anti-microbial and anti-inflammatory therapy for cystic fibrosis. Paediatr Respir Rev. 2014;15(2):154–62.
14. Black PN, Scragg R. Relationship between serum 25-hydroxyvitamin d and pulmonary function in the third national health and nutrition examination survey. Chest. 2005;128(6):3792–8.
15. McCauley LA, Thomas W, Laguna TA, Regelmann WE, Moran A, Polgreen LE. Vitamin D deficiency is associated with pulmonary exacerbations in children with cystic fibrosis. Ann Am Thorac Soc. 2014;11(2):198–204.
16. Wolfenden LL, Judd SE, Shah R, Sanyal R, Ziegler TR, Tangpricha V. Vitamin D and bone health in adults with cystic fibrosis. Clin Endocrinol. 2008;69(3):374–81.
17. Grossmann RE, Zughaier SM, Kumari M, Seydafkan S, Lyles RH, Liu S, et al. Pilot study of vitamin D supplementation in adults with cystic fibrosis pulmonary exacerbation: a randomized, controlled trial. Dermatoendocrinology. 2012;4(2):191–7.
18. Hewison M. Vitamin D, and the intracrinology of innate immunity. Mol Cell Endocrinol. 2010;321(2):103–11.
19. Yim S, Dhawan P, Ragunath C, Christakos S, Diamond G. Induction of cathelicidin in normal and CF bronchial epithelial cells by 1,25-dihydroxyvitamin D(3). J Cyst Fibros. 2007;6(6):403–10.
20. Kassey H, Nurlan D, Julie B, Simon R, Larry L. Supplementation with 25-hydroxyvitamin D3 down-regulates pathogen-stimulated interleukin-8 production in cystic fibrosis macrophages and airway epithelial cells. B35

pathogenesis and clinical issues in cystic fibrosis. Am Thorac Soc Int Conf Abstr. 2012;A2803-A.
21. Grossmann RE, Zughaier SM, Liu S, Lyles RH, Tangpricha V. Impact of vitamin D supplementation on markers of inflammation in adults with cystic fibrosis hospitalized for a pulmonary exacerbation. Eur J Clin Nutr. 2012;66(9):1072–4.
22. Tangpricha V, Kelly A, Stephenson A, Maguiness K, Enders J, Robinson KA, et al. An update on the screening, diagnosis, management, and treatment of vitamin D deficiency in individuals with cystic fibrosis: evidence-based recommendations from the cystic fibrosis foundation. J Clin Endocrinol Metab. 2012;97(4):1082–93.
23. Chandra P, Wolfenden LL, Ziegler TR, Tian J, Luo M, Stecenko AA, et al. Treatment of vitamin D deficiency with UV light in patients with malabsorption syndromes: a case series. Photodermatol Photoimmunol Photomed. 2007;23(5):179–85.
24. Khazai NB, Judd SE, Jeng L, Wolfenden LL, Stecenko A, Ziegler TR, et al. Treatment and prevention of vitamin D insufficiency in cystic fibrosis patients: comparative efficacy of ergocalciferol, cholecalciferol, and UV light. J Clin Endocrinol Metab. 2009;94(6):2037–43.
25. Gronowitz E, Larko O, Gilljam M, Hollsing A, Lindblad A, Mellstrom D, et al. Ultraviolet B radiation improves serum levels of vitamin D in patients with cystic fibrosis. Acta Paediatr. 2005;94(5):547–52. Oslo, Norway: 1992.

Chapter 4
Vitamin D Deficiency in Anorexia Nervosa

Supavit Chesdachai and Vin Tangpricha

Case Presentation

A 28-year-old Caucasian woman with anorexia nervosa was referred to endocrinology clinic for evaluation of osteoporosis and vitamin D deficiency. Two months prior to this visit, she had been hospitalized for hypokalemia, hypomagnesemia, hypophosphatemia, and metabolic alkalosis, which were due to severe vomiting from anorexia nervosa/bulimia. She was also found to have very low bone density and vitamin D deficiency. Her bone mineral density (BMD) was lower than the normal young adult. T-score at spine was less than −2.0 and hip was less than −2.5 which was in

S. Chesdachai, M.D. (✉)
Mahidol University, Bangkok, Thailand
e-mail: s.chesdachai@gmail.com

V. Tangpricha, M.D., Ph.D.
Emory University School of Medicine, Atlanta, GA, USA
e-mail: vin.tangpricha@emory.edu

© Springer International Publishing Switzerland 2016
V. Tangpricha (ed.), *Vitamin D*,
DOI 10.1007/978-3-319-26176-8_4

osteoporosis range. Her serum 25-hydroxyvitamin D (25(OH)D) was 17 ng/mL. Her parathyroid hormone level (PTH) was 7 pg/mL which was low. She received 50,000 IU of ergocalciferol (vitamin D_2) daily for 2 weeks during hospitalization to improve her vitamin D status.

She had been struggling with her eating disorder for over 15 years. Her weight has been stable over the past years; her body mass index (BMI) was 17.3 kg/m^2. She had poor appetite and previously reported self-induced emesis at least once a day. Her menstrual period was irregular. She had been hospitalized in the past for abnormal liver function tests and severe malnutrition. She took escitalopram and many nutrient supplements for her condition. She did not eat any diary products, fish, or egg yolks. She had history of traumatic fracture at her right arm in the past but she denies any bone pain or muscle ache. Her family members were all in good state of health. Her physical examinations were within normal limits.

Diagnosis and Assessment

This patient presented with anorexia nervosa, osteoporosis, and vitamin D deficiency. The etiology of vitamin D deficiency in patients with anorexia nervosa is in part due to insufficient dietary intake of vitamin D-containing foods and supplements.

Low bone density, and osteoporosis in patients with anorexia nervosa are related to many factors. Alteration of body composition, low BMI, and decrease lean body mass are associated with low bone density [1, 2]. Severe malnutrition leads to disturbance of many hormonal axes such as hypogonadism, relativel hypercortisolemia, and growth hormone resistance [3]. Other causes that can also affect bone density are inadequate calcium intake, long term selective serotonin reuptake inhibitors (SSRIs) intake, and vitamin D deficiency [2, 3].

Management

According to the Endocrine Society 2011 Clinical Practice Guidelines on Vitamin D [4], patients with vitamin D deficiency should be treated with 50,000 IU of ergocalciferol (vitamin D_2) or cholecalciferol (vitamin D_3) once a week for 8 weeks or 6000 IU daily. Then 1500–2000 IU vitamin D daily is needed as a maintenance therapy to keep serum 25(OH)D above 30 ng/mL (75 nmol/L). In order to maintain adequate vitamin D status, she should increase intake of vitamin D-containing foods such as fortified diary products, oily fish, mushrooms, or egg yolks and increase sunlight exposure.

Treatment of osteopenia and osteoporosis in patients with anorexia nervosa is challenging. A systematic review of randomized controlled trials demonstrates that bisphosphonate and estrogen therapy showed no benefit. Weight restoration and improving of nutritional status may play a role in the treatment of osteopenia and osteoporosis [5].

Outcome

At the clinic, her total serum 25(OH)D concentration reaches 30 ng/mL after 2 weeks of daily ergocalciferol. She is taking 1200 mg calcium and 1500 IU of vitamin D per day. She is followed every 6 months in clinic to monitor her BMD and vitamin D status to ensure adequate nutritional status.

Discussion and Literature Review

Anorexia nervosa is a common eating disorder in female adolescents and young women. It is characterized by fear of weight gain, body-image disturbance, and food intake restriction leading to severe weight loss and many organic complications [6, 7]. Incidence and prevalence of anorexia nervosa is highest in female adolescent between 15 and 19 years of age. The overall incidence is up to 8 per 100,000 people [8, 9] and the prevalence is 0.9 % in adult female [9]. According to one meta-analysis, mortality rate of anorexia nervosa is approximately 5.25 % per decade [10].

Complications of anorexia nervosa are mainly from starvation that leads to malfunction of many organ systems. Electrolyte imbalance and cardiovascular complications are the leading causes of death [11, 12]. Low bone density is a common complication in anorexia nervosa. More than 50 % of patients with anorexia nervosa have osteopenia [13] and lifetime prevalence of fracture is 60 % higher than normal population [14]. Cross-sectional studies demonstrated that Z-scores from lumbar spine, hip, and femoral neck for adolescent girls with anorexia nervosa are significantly lower than healthy controls [15, 16].

Vitamin D regulates intestinal calcium and phosphorus absorption. Low vitamin D level leads to decreased bone mineralization and increased risk of fracture, osteopenia, and osteoporosis [17]. One large cohort of patients with anorexia nervosa without vitamin D supplementation demonstrated a strong positive correlation between vitamin D status and BMD [18]. A recent cross-sectional study demonstrates that prevalence of vitamin D insufficiency and deficiency in patients with anorexia nervosa is 23 % and 8 %, respectively.

However, several studies found that there was no difference in serum 25(OH)D between the patients with anorexia nervosa and healthy controls [19–21]. Haagensen *et al.* demonstrate that prevalence of vitamin D deficiency was 2 % in patients with anorexia nervosa compared with 24 % in healthy controls [22]. These finding may be due to decreased fat storage of vitamin D leading to higher serum 25(OH)D, decreased metabolic clearance, and effective vitamin D supplementation [22, 23].

Anorexia nervosa can also occur with other psychiatric morbidities such as mood disorder, anxiety disorder, obsessive compulsive disorder, and alcohol or substance abuse [6]. Increase rates of suicide from depression and alcohol abuse are one of the causes of death in anorexia nervosa aside from the other medical complications [10]. Systematic reviews and meta-analyses have demonstrated that low vitamin D status is associated with depression [24, 25] and that vitamin D supplementation may help improve depression in anorexia nervosa patients [26].

Effective vitamin D supplementation is important to maintain sufficient vitamin D status in patients with anorexia nervosa. A prospective, experimental pilot study demonstrated that oral bioavailability of high-dose ergocalciferol in patients with anorexia nervosa and healthy controls are the same [23]. Moreover, meta-analysis from four cross-sectional studies shows that serum 25(OH)D in patients with anorexia without vitamin D supplementation is significantly lower than healthy controls. In contrast, serum 25(OH)D concentrations are significantly higher in patients with anorexia nervosa that receive vitamin D supplementation [27]. In conclusion, serum 25(OH)D should be tested in patients with anorexia nervosa to determine vitamin D status. Low vitamin D status should be treated according to the Endocrine Society's 2011 Clinical Practice Guidelines on Vitamin D.

Clinical Pearls and Pitfalls

- Vitamin D deficiency is common in patients with anorexia nervosa.
- Low vitamin D status is associated with low bone density, osteopenia, and osteoporosis in patients with anorexia nervosa.
- Serum 25(OH)D should be tested in patients with anorexia nervosa to determine vitamin D status and should be maintained at least 30 ng/mL.
- Effective vitamin D supplementation is important to maintain sufficient 25(OH)D concentrations in patients with anorexia nervosa.

Suggested Reading

1. Veronese N, Solmi M, Rizza W, Manzato E, Sergi G, Santonastaso P, et al. Vitamin D status in anorexia nervosa: a meta-analysis. Int J Eat Disord. 2014.
2. Holick MF, Binkley NC, Bischoff-Ferrari HA, Gordon CM, Hanley DA, Heaney RP, et al. Evaluation, treatment, and

prevention of vitamin D deficiency: an endocrine society clinical practice guideline. J Clin Endocrinol Metab. 2011; 96(7):1911–30.

References

1. Miller KK, Lee EE, Lawson EA, Misra M, Minihan J, Grinspoon SK, et al. Determinants of skeletal loss and recovery in anorexia nervosa. J Clin Endocrinol Metab. 2006;91(8):2931–7.
2. Misra M, Klibanski A. Bone metabolism in adolescents with anorexia nervosa. J Endocrinol Investig. 2011;34(4):324–32.
3. Misra M, Klibanski A. Bone health in anorexia nervosa. Curr Opin Endocrinol Diabetes Obes. 2011;18(6):376–82.
4. Holick MF, Binkley NC, Bischoff-Ferrari HA, Gordon CM, Hanley DA, Heaney RP, et al. Evaluation, treatment, and prevention of vitamin D deficiency: an endocrine society clinical practice guideline. J Clin Endocrinol Metab. 2011;96(7):1911–30.
5. Mehler PS, MacKenzie TD. Treatment of osteopenia and osteoporosis in anorexia nervosa: a systematic review of the literature. Int J Eat Disord. 2009;42(3):195–201.
6. Yager J, Andersen AE. Clinical practice. Anorexia nervosa. N Engl J Med. 2005;353(14):1481–8.
7. American Psychiatric Association. Diagnostic and statistical manual of mental disorders (DSM-5®). Washington, DC: American Psychiatric Association; 2013.
8. Hoek HW. Incidence, prevalence and mortality of anorexia nervosa and other eating disorders. Curr Opin Psychiatry. 2006;19(4): 389–94.
9. Smink FR, van Hoeken D, Hoek HW. Epidemiology of eating disorders: incidence, prevalence and mortality rates. Curr Psychiatry Rep. 2012;14(4):406–14.
10. Signorini A, De Filippo E, Panico S, De Caprio C, Pasanisi F, Contaldo F. Long-term mortality in anorexia nervosa: a report after an 8-year follow-up and a review of the most recent literature. Eur J Clin Nutr. 2007;61(1):119–22.
11. Golden NH. Eating disorders in adolescence and their sequelae. Best Pract Res Clin Obstet Gynaecol. 2003;17(1):57–73.
12. Mehler PS, Brown C. Anorexia nervosa – medical complications. J Eat Disord. 2015;3:11.
13. Munoz MT, Argente J. Anorexia nervosa in female adolescents: endocrine and bone mineral density disturbances. Eur J Endocrinol. 2002; 147(3):275–86.

14. Faje AT, Fazeli PK, Miller KK, Katzman DK, Ebrahimi S, Lee H, et al. Fracture risk and areal bone mineral density in adolescent females with anorexia nervosa. Int J Eat Disord. 2014;47(5):458–66.

15. Misra M, Aggarwal A, Miller KK, Almazan C, Worley M, Soyka LA, et al. Effects of anorexia nervosa on clinical, hematologic, biochemical, and bone density parameters in community-dwelling adolescent girls. Pediatrics. 2004;114(6):1574–83.

16. Soyka LA, Misra M, Frenchman A, Miller KK, Grinspoon S, Schoenfeld DA, et al. Abnormal bone mineral accrual in adolescent girls with anorexia nervosa. J Clin Endocrinol Metab. 2002;87(9):4177–85.

17. Holick MF. Vitamin D, deficiency. N Engl J Med. 2007;357 (3):266–81.

18. Gatti D, El Ghoch M, Viapiana O, Ruocco A, Chignola E, Rossini M, et al. Strong relationship between vitamin D status and bone mineral density in anorexia nervosa. Bone. 2015;78:212–5.

19. Olmos JM, Riancho JA, Amado JA, Freijanes J, Menendez-Arango J, Gonzalez-Macias J. Vitamin D metabolism and serum binding proteins in anorexia nervosa. Bone. 1991;12(1):43–6.

20. Van Binsbergen CJ, Odink J, Van den Berg H, Koppeschaar H, Coelingh Bennink HJ. Nutritional status in anorexia nervosa: clinical chemistry, vitamins, iron and zinc. Eur J Clin Nutr. 1988;42(11):929–37.

21. Aarskog D, Aksnes L, Markestad T, Trygstad O. Plasma concentrations of vitamin D metabolites in pubertal girls with anorexia nervosa. Acta Endocrinol Suppl (Copenh). 1986;279:458–67.

22. Haagensen AL, Feldman HA, Ringelheim J, Gordon CM. Low prevalence of vitamin D deficiency among adolescents with anorexia nervosa. Osteoporos Int. 2008;19(3):289–94.

23. Divasta AD, Feldman HA, Brown JN, Giancaterino C, Holick MF, Gordon CM. Bioavailability of vitamin D in malnourished adolescents with anorexia nervosa. J Clin Endocrinol Metab. 2011;96(8):2575–80.

24. Ju SY, Lee YJ, Jeong SN. Serum 25-hydroxyvitamin D levels and the risk of depression: a systematic review and meta-analysis. J Nutr Health Aging. 2013;17(5):447–55.

25. Anglin RE, Samaan Z, Walter SD, McDonald SD. Vitamin D deficiency and depression in adults: systematic review and meta-analysis. Br J Psychiatry. 2013;202:100–7.

26. Spedding S. Vitamin D, and depression: a systematic review and meta-analysis comparing studies with and without biological flaws. Nutrients. 2014;6(4):1501–18.

27. Veronese N, Solmi M, Rizza W, Manzato E, Sergi G, Santonastaso P, et al. Vitamin D status in anorexia nervosa: a meta-analysis. Int J Eat Disord. 2014.

Chapter 5
Vitamin D Deficiency Following Bariatric Surgery

Malcolm D. Kearns and Vin Tangpricha

Case Presentation

A 46-year-old female who underwent bariatric surgery 4 years ago presented in clinic for an evaluation of vitamin D deficiency, hyperparathyroidism, and bone loss. The surgery was a biliopancreatic diversion, a procedure in which the small bowel was resected and the terminal ilium connected to a short section of proximal duodenum. Following the procedure, the patient achieved a 160-pound weight loss. However, 6 months later, the patient developed severe vitamin D deficiency that did not respond to vitamin D repletion (50,000 IU of vitamin D given once a week followed by 50,000 IU of vitamin D per month). A bone mineral density (BMD) scan

M.D. Kearns, M.D. (✉)
University of Pennsylvania,
3400 Spruce St, Philadelphia, PA 19104, USA
e-mail: malcolmdkearns@gmail.com

V. Tangpricha, M.D., Ph.D.
Emory University School of Medicine, Atlanta, GA, USA
e-mail: vin.tangpricha@emory.edu

© Springer International Publishing Switzerland 2016
V. Tangpricha (ed.), *Vitamin D*,
DOI 10.1007/978-3-319-26176-8_5

performed 2 years following the surgery showed osteopenia, particularly in the spine and right trochanter. Laboratory values at that time showed serum 25-hydroxyvitamin D (25(OH)D) concentration to be low (18 ng/mL) in spite of vitamin D supplementation and parathyroid hormone (PTH) to be elevated to 71 pg/mL (laboratory range: 10–65 pg/mL). In the year prior to her presentation, she began having irregular menstruations and was determined to be in menopause by elevated follicle-stimulating hormone (FSH). She also began experiencing bone pain in her right hip and shin. Her daily medication regimen at presentation included a multivitamin, which included the fat-soluble vitamins A, D, E, and K, 600 mg of calcium citrate t.i.d., and zinc supplements. She continued to receive a 50,000 IU dose of vitamin D each month.

Diagnosis/Assessment

Labs drawn at the time of presentation showed very low serum 25(OH)D concentration (<7 ng/mL), elevated PTH concentration (177 pg/mL), and normal serum 1,25 dihydroxyvitamin D (1,25(OH)$_2$D), calcium, and phosphorous. The history of bone pain and low BMD following bariatric surgery coupled with low vitamin D status and elevated PTH concentration was consistent with the diagnosis of vitamin D deficiency accompanied by secondary hyperparathyroidism. The mechanism of this presentation is largely due to gut malabsorption, which is a major cause of weight loss in bariatric surgery. The small bowel is essential for absorbing calcium and fat-soluble vitamins, including vitamin D. However, although low vitamin D alone can lead to secondary hyperparathyroidism, only 30 % of patients diagnosed with secondary hyperparathyroidism following bariatric surgery are vitamin D deficient [1]. Thus, low calcium absorption in the gut is also likely contributory to the secondary hyperparathyroidism. Though calcium absorption is dramatically reduced following removal of the duodenum and jejunum, hypocalcemia is rare following bariatric surgery [2] since an elevated PTH concentration PTH typically maintains normal calcium concentration at the expense of bone health.

Management

The initial treatment of vitamin D deficiency and hyperparathyroidism involves aggressive supplementation with vitamin D and calcium. The effects of treatment on bone health can be followed on annual bone mineral density scans by dual X-ray absorptiometry (DEXA). Following her presentation, this patient received a vitamin D load with 50,000 IU/day of vitamin D for 10 days along with 3000 mg of calcium per day. After 2 months, her laboratory values appeared to respond; her serum 25(OH)D concentration increased to 28 ng/mL and her calcium and phosphorous remained within normal limits. However, her PTH concentration remained elevated (91 pg/mL).

She continued on vitamin D (50,000 IU of vitamin D twice a week with 3000 mg calcium per day) in order to maintain serum 25(OH)D concentration >30 ng/mL. However, on follow-up visit, her 25(OH)D concentration dropped to 22 ng/mL and her PTH increased to 180 pg/mL in spite of the high-dose maintenance vitamin D. The next step in therapy involved adding activated vitamin D in the form of calcitriol (0.5 mcg b.i.d.) with the aim of increasing gut absorption of calcium and decreasing PTH concentration. The addition of this therapy was accompanied with a 24-h urine collection to assess for her ability to absorb calcium and to ensure she was not having hypercalciuria.

Following the addition of calcitriol, this patient's regimen was eventually modified to 4000 mg of elemental calcium per day in divided doses, calcitriol 0.5 mcg orally twice daily and 50,000 IU of cholecalciferol orally four times per week. This regimen brought the patient's PTH levels down into the normal range, though she had difficulty consistently maintaining serum 25(OH)D >30 ng/mL.

In spite of this intensive therapy, her serial BMD scans continued to show bone loss. Adding a bisphosphonate, to reduce bone resorption by blocking the action of osteoclasts, was considered. However, it was determined that the cause of this patient's hyperparathyroidism may largely be linked to poor intestinal absorption of calcium. Thus, if the bones are her primary source of calcium, inhibiting bone resorption with a bisphosphonate would increase her risk of hypocalcemia.

Outcome

In spite continually increasing doses of vitamin D and calcium, providing oral calcitriol, and ultimately suppressing the patient's PTH concentration, the patient continued to have bone loss. She developed osteopenia (*T*-score between −1.0 and −2.5) prior to her presentation and eventually osteoporosis (*T*-score < −2.5) after 2 years of treatment on the above regimen. Though she fortunately experienced no fractures up to this point, her spine, left hip, and right hip had lost 22 %, 16.8 %, and 15.3 % of their BMD, respectively, compared to her initial BMD test. Ultimately, 5 years following the presentation described above, the patient continued to be vitamin D deficient (8 ng/mL) though $1,25(OH)_2D$ and PTH were within normal limits. In the setting of continually worsening bone density, the patient was started on an anabolic bone agent (teriparatide at 20 mcg daily for 2 years). Such agents can be used in the short term to increase bone density. With the addition of an anabolic bone agent, the patient's BMD measurements stabilized the following year. The patient moved shortly after and began to receive care at a different institution.

Discussion and Literature Review

Abnormalities in vitamin D metabolism, calcium absorption, and PTH concentration are common surrounding bariatric surgery. Even before surgery, obese individuals have lower serum vitamin D and higher PTH concentrations than age- and gender-matched subjects [3]. However, while obesity typically protects against osteoporosis, the dramatic weight loss associated with bariatric surgery increases the risk for low bone mass and metabolic bone disease [4–6]. One study showed BMD to decrease by 7.8 % in the hips, 9.3 % in the trochanters, and 1.6 % in the total body in the 9 months following surgery [4]. While reduced mechanical unloading likely contributes to bone loss, malabsorption of nutrients in the gut is likely the primary etiology. Removal of the small intestines reduces the surface over which vitamin D is absorbed, and up to 80 % of dietary calcium is absorbed in the duodenum and proximal jejunum [2]. As a result of decreased vitamin D and calcium absorption, PTH concentration tends to be increased following bariatric surgeries; in one study, mean PTH levels more than doubled in 1 year following bariatric surgery [7], and in another study, over 50 % of morbidly obese women had PTH above the normal range within 2 years following surgery [1]. Factors that place individuals at risk for hyperparathyroidism following surgery include age (menopause likely exacerbates bone resorption), higher BMI prior to surgery, and race (African–Americans experience significantly more hyperparathyroidism following surgery than Caucasian patients [1]). The likelihood of elevated PTH following surgery is also related to the amount of malabsorption in the procedure done. While 30–50% of patients may have elevated PTH following a gastric bypass, the more malabsorptive biliopancreatic diversion leads to 50–80 % of individuals having elevated PTH [8].

Elevated PTH can have negative effects on bone mineral density. Thus initial treatment following bariatric surgery should involve aggressive supplementation with calcium and vitamin D. Studies show daily vitamin D doses of 2000 or 5000 IU [9] and weekly doses of 50,000 IU [10] are often necessary to prevent bone disease following bariatric surgery. However, as demonstrated by this case, higher doses may be required in some patients. Providing adequate calcium supplementation is also essential following malabsorptive procedures. Daily calcium doses should typically be 1200–1500 mg after gastric bypass surgery and 2000 mg after duodenal switch [11, 12], though higher doses may be necessary in some patients. Calcium citrate is the preferred formulation, exhibiting better intestinal absorption than calcium carbonate [13], though calcium citrate is often more expensive and requires larger capsules than calcium carbonate.

If additional measures are needed to suppress PTH, calcitriol decreases the synthesis of PTH at the RNA level [14], increases calcium absorption directly in the intestines, and increases the sensitivity of calcium-sensing receptors in the parathyroid glands in suppressing PTH release. Bisphosphonates can also be added to reduce bone resorption. However, these medications should be used with extreme caution to guard against hypocalcemia given that bisphosphonates will inhibit osteoclast function and reduce the release of calcium mineral from the bone. One study demonstrated that alendronate, a bisphosphonate, was effective in improving BMD of the lumbar spine in individuals who did not show improvement with several years of vitamin D therapy alone following a gastrectomy [15]. As demonstrated in this case, anabolic bone agents may also be used temporarily in the setting of continued bone loss. However, the effect of anabolic agents on fracture risk is unknown.

Clinical Pearls/Pitfalls

- Malabsorption of macro- and micronutrients commonly occurs following gastric bypass surgery. It is important to be aware of the possibility for vitamin deficiencies and metabolic bone disease following surgery.
- Symptoms of metabolic bone disease following bariatric surgery often include bone pain.
- Treatment for vitamin D deficiency and secondary hyperparathyroidism should begin with optimizing vitamin D status and providing daily calcium supplements.
- Adding the activated form of vitamin D, calcitriol, can be used if vitamin D status cannot be optimized through oral supplementation.
- Bisphosphonate therapy should be used with caution in individuals with osteoporosis secondary to malabsorption, since these individuals have increased risk of hypocalcemia.
- Hypocalcemia is rare following gastric bypass. Though calcium absorption is dramatically reduced following removal of the duodenum and jejunum, PTH typically maintains normal calcium concentration at the expense of bone health.

Suggested Reading

1. Coates PS, Fernstrom JD, Fernstrom MH, Schauer PR, Greenspan SL. Gastric bypass surgery for morbid obesity leads to an increase in bone turnover and a decrease in bone mass. J Clin Endocrinol Metab. 2004;89(3):1061–5.
2. Heber D, Greenway FL, Kaplan LM, Livingston E, Salvador J, Still C, et al. Endocrine and nutritional management of the post-bariatric surgery patient: an endocrine society clinical practice guideline. J Clin Endocrinol Metab. 2010;95(11):4823–43.

References

1. Youssef Y, Richards WO, Sekhar N, Kaiser J, Spagnoli A, Abumrad N, et al. Risk of secondary hyperparathyroidism after laparoscopic gastric bypass surgery in obese women. Surg Endosc. 2007;21(8):1393–6.
2. Carlin AM, Rao DS, Yager KM, Genaw JA, Parikh NJ, Szymanski W. Effect of gastric bypass surgery on vitamin D nutritional status. Surg Obes Relat Dis. 2006;2(6):638–42.
3. Snijder MB, van Dam RM, Visser M, Deeg DJ, Dekker JM, Bouter LM, et al. Adiposity in relation to vitamin D status and parathyroid hormone levels: a population-based study in older men and women. J Clin Endocrinol Metab. 2005;90(7):4119–23.
4. Coates PS, Fernstrom JD, Fernstrom MH, Schauer PR, Greenspan SL. Gastric bypass surgery for morbid obesity leads to an increase in bone turnover and a decrease in bone mass. J Clin Endocrinol Metab. 2004;89(3):1061–5.
5. Bano G, Rodin DA, Pazianas M, Nussey SS. Reduced bone mineral density after surgical treatment for obesity. Int J Obes Relat Metab Disord. 1999;23(4):361–5.
6. Crowley LV, Seay J, Mullin G. Late effects of gastric bypass for obesity. Am J Gastroenterol. 1984;79(11):850–60.
7. Jin J, Robinson AV, Hallowell PT, Jasper JJ, Stellato TA, Wilhem SM. Increases in parathyroid hormone (PTH) after gastric bypass surgery appear to be of a secondary nature. Surgery. 2007;142(6):914–20. discussion 914–20.
8. Hewitt S, Sovik TT, Aasheim ET, Kristinsson J, Jahnsen J, Birketvedt GS, et al. Secondary hyperparathyroidism, vitamin D sufficiency, and serum calcium 5 years after gastric bypass and duodenal switch. Obes Surg. 2013;23(3):384–90.

9. Goldner WS, Stoner JA, Lyden E, Thompson J, Taylor K, Larson L, et al. Finding the optimal dose of vitamin D following Roux-en-Y gastric bypass: a prospective, randomized pilot clinical trial. Obes Surg. 2009;19(2):173–9.

10. Carlin AM, Rao DS, Yager KM, Parikh NJ, Kapke A. Treatment of vitamin D depletion after Roux-en-Y gastric bypass: a randomized prospective clinical trial. Surg Obes Relat Dis. 2009;5(4):444–9.

11. Heber D, Greenway FL, Kaplan LM, Livingston E, Salvador J, Still C, et al. Endocrine and nutritional management of the post-bariatric surgery patient: an endocrine society clinical practice guideline. J Clin Endocrinol Metab. 2010;95(11):4823–43.

12. Mechanick JI, Kushner RF, Sugerman HJ, Gonzalez-Campoy JM, Collazo-Clavell ML, Spitz AF, et al. American Association of Clinical Endocrinologists, The Obesity Society, and American Society for Metabolic and Bariatric Surgery medical guidelines for clinical practice for the perioperative nutritional, metabolic, and nonsurgical support of the bariatric surgery patient. Obesity. 2009;17 Suppl 1:S1–70. v.

13. Tondapu P, Provost D, Adams-Huet B, Sims T, Chang C, Sakhaee K. Comparison of the absorption of calcium carbonate and calcium citrate after Roux-en-Y gastric bypass. Obes Surg. 2009;19(9):1256–61.

14. Silver J, Russell J, Sherwood LM. Regulation by vitamin D metabolites of messenger ribonucleic acid for preproparathyroid hormone in isolated bovine parathyroid cells. Proc Natl Acad Sci U S A. 1985;82(12):4270–3.

15. Suzuki Y, Ishibashi Y, Omura N, Kawasaki N, Kashiwagi H, Yanaga K, et al. Alendronate improves vitamin D-resistant osteopenia triggered by gastrectomy in patients with gastric cancer followed long term. J Gastrointest Surg. 2005;9(7):955–60.

Chapter 6
Vitamin D in Postsurgical Hypoparathyroidism

Maria Lee and Vin Tangpricha

Case Presentation

A 46-year-old Caucasian female with a 20-year history of toxic multinodular goiter presented with complaints of thyroid growth, anterior neck discomfort, intermittent dysphagia, sensation of pressure when lying supine, and intermittently scratchy voice. She had taken methimazole on and off for twenty years and had had numerous ultrasounds and fine needle aspirates over the years. Her other medical problems included severe gastroesophageal reflux disease, transient ischemic attack, and nephrolithiasis; surgeries included

M. Lee, M.D. (✉)
Emory University School of Medicine, 1303 Woodruff Memorial Research Building, 101 Woodruff Circle, Suite 1303, Atlanta, GA 30322, USA
e-mail: mnlee2@emory.edu

V. Tangpricha, M.D., Ph.D.
Emory University School of Medicine, Atlanta, GA, USA
e-mail: vin.tangpricha@emory.edu

© Springer International Publishing Switzerland 2016
V. Tangpricha (ed.), *Vitamin D*,
DOI 10.1007/978-3-319-26176-8_6

41

cholecystectomy and hysterectomy. Family history was notable for hyperthyroidism resulting in thyroidectomy in her nieces and one of her daughters as well as hyperthyroidism in her paternal grandmother. She was a 20-pack-year smoker but did not drink alcohol or use illicit drugs. The patient recently had a fine needle aspirate performed on a right thyroid nodule that was reported to be 2.48 cm, mixed solid-cystic (mostly solid), hypoechoic with internal calcifications and increased vascularity on ultrasound which returned benign on cytology. She also had a 2.24 cm thyroid nodule that met criteria for FNA, but she did not tolerate the procedure long enough to undergo biopsy of this nodule. A thyroid uptake scan showed homogeneous increased uptake consistent with Graves' disease and a cold nodule in the right thyroid lobe. After discussion with an endocrinologist and a general surgeon, she decided to undergo thyroidectomy to relieve the compressive symptoms as well as rule out malignancy.

Diagnosis and Assessment

The patient underwent total thyroidectomy. The right upper and left upper parathyroid glands were sought but could not be found. The right lower and left lower parathyroid glands were identified but could not be spared in situ, so they were each autografted. Preoperatively, the patient's corrected calcium level was 9.1. The evening after the surgery, the corrected calcium dropped to 7.94 and phosphorus elevated at 5.0 with PTH<6 (undetectable). This patient developed hypocalcemia and hyperphosphatemia due to iatrogenic or postsurgical hypoparathyroidism, as confirmed by the undetectable PTH level postoperatively.

Management

The patient was started on calcitriol 0.25 mcg twice a day and calcium-vitamin D 500 mg–200 units 2 tabs three times a day. The corrected calcium down-trended the next day to 7.4 so the dose of calcitriol was increased to 0.5 mcg twice a day. On post-op day 2, the corrected calcium was 9.3, phosphorus 4.3, PTH still undetectable, and the patient was discharged on a regimen of calcitriol 0.25 mcg twice a day and calcium-vitamin D 500 mg–200 units 2 tabs three times a day with recommendations to recheck calcium, phosphorus, albumin, and PTH a few days after discharge. The results of these labs are unknown because she followed up with her primary care physician and endocrinologist at a different facility. The pathology of the total thyroidectomy specimens returned as multinodular follicular hyperplasia.

Discussion and Literature Review

Parathyroid cells sense a reduction in serum ionized calcium and respond by stimulating release of parathyroid hormone, which increases bone resorption, increases calcium reabsorption from the distal convoluted tubules in the kidneys, and decreases reabsorption of phosphorus from the proximal convoluted tubules. It also stimulates 1-alpha-hydroxylase activity in the kidney, leading to increased conversion of 25-hydroxyvitamin D_3 to 1,25-dihydroxyvitamin D_3 [1].

Hypoparathyroidism is a condition in which the parathyroid gland does not produce enough parathyroid hormone (true hypoparathyroidism) or when the target tissue (bone, kidneys) becomes resistant to the action of the parathyroid hormone (pseudohypoparathyroidism). As opposed to other etiologies such as autoimmune disorders, genetic syndromes, infiltrative diseases, etc., postsurgical hypoparathyroidism is a result of accidental removal, devascularization, or manipulation of the parathyroid glands during thyroidectomy, parathyroidectomy, or neck surgery for head and neck cancer. Biochemically it is characterized by hypocalcemia, hyperphosphatemia or high normal serum phosphorus, and low PTH levels within hours after surgery. Transient hypoparathyroidism is seen in about 10 % of patients who undergo total thyroidectomy. Most patients recover parathyroid function within 6 months of thyroid surgery, but a small percentage (4.4 %) develop permanent hypoparathyroidism, defined as the requirement of medical treatment for longer than 12 months. Risk factors for postsurgical hypoparathyroidism include low calcium levels before surgery, failure to identify all the parathyroid glands during surgery, pregnancy, lactation, and parathyroid autotransplantation, while bilateral central ligation of the inferior thyroid artery and thyroidectomy for a highly vascularized goiter (e.g., Graves' disease), recurrent goiter, or extensive lymph node dissection for thyroid cancer increase the chance of permanent hypoparathyroidism [1]. Hypoparathyroidism after parathyroidectomy is rarer and occurs in less than 1 % of initial surgery for primary hyperparathyroidism but does increase up to 30 % after surgeries for recurrent or persistent hyperparathyroidism. Transient hypocalcemia after parathyroidectomy usually does not require treatment unless severe or symptomatic, unlike severe or prolonged hypocalcemia due to hungry bone syndrome, in which there is a significant increase in bone formation and resultant hypocalcemia and hypophosphatemia.

Diagnosis of hypoparathyroidism involves biochemical findings of hypocalcemia, hyperphosphatemia or high normal serum phosphorus, and low PTH levels and sometimes clinical symptoms as well. Pooled data from nine studies showed that a greater than 65 % decline in PTH level from baseline to 6 h after surgery had the greatest accuracy in predicting hypocalcemia, with 96.4 % sensitivity and 91.4 % specificity; therefore it is recommended to check these levels 6 h postoperatively, especially since some patients may be asymptomatic initially [2]. Clinical manifestations of hypoparathyroidism depend upon the severity of hypocalcemia and rapidity of onset. Milder symptoms include paresthesias of the distal extremities or around the mouth, carpopedal spasm, and twitching/cramping, while severe symptoms range from confusion, seizure, laryngospasm, bronchospasm to congestive heart failure and arrhythmias due to a prolonged QT interval. Hypocalcemia can sometimes be detected on physical exam with the Chvostek sign, in which tapping on the facial nerve elicits contraction of ipsilateral facial muscles, or Trousseau sign, where inflation of a blood pressure cuff for several minutes leads to wrist flexion, interphalangeal joint extension, and thumb adduction.

Immediate management of postsurgical hypoparathyroidism involves oral supplementation with elemental calcium 1–2 g three times daily and calcitriol 0.25–1 mcg two or three times daily. In patients with or at risk of severe hypocalcemia, elemental calcium is started at 2 g three times daily and calcitriol 0.5 mcg three times daily. For patients with corrected serum calcium levels less than 7.5 mg/dL or with acute symptoms of hypocalcemia, it is recommended to start a continuous 10 % calcium gluconate drip along with oral supplementation. The drip may be continued until the oral therapy becomes effectively absorbed; serum calcium should be monitored frequently (e.g., every 6–8 h), depending on the patient's symptoms and severity of hypocalcemia. The oral/intravenous calcium dosages should be titrated according to a target serum calcium level 8.0–8.5 mg/dL. Concomitant vitamin D deficiency and hypomagnesemia should also be treated since vitamin D deficiency can lead to significant hypocalcemia, and hypomagnesemia contributes to PTH resistance. In January 2015, recombinant human PTH (Natpara) was approved in the United States as an adjunct to calcium and calcitriol to treat hypocalcemia in patients with hypoparathyroidism; it has the potential to normalize defective bone metabolism and achieve normal calcium levels without causing hypercalciuria and other complications seen with high doses of calcium and calcitriol [3]. In one case report, post-thyroidectomy hypoparathyroidism unresponsive to oral calcium, magnesium, and high-dose calcitriol was successfully treated with multipulse subcutaneous infusion of teriparatide, but it is not commonly used in clinical practice at this time [4].

According to the American Association of Clinical Endocrinologists and American College of Endocrinology, intraoperative PTH levels can expedite same-day discharge or predict the need for observation and postoperative calcium management. Patients with PTH greater than 15 ng/mL measured 20 min or longer after surgery can be discharged home on prophylactic calcium. Patients with PTH less than 15 ng/mL should be started on calcitriol, calcium, and possibly magnesium and observed overnight [5]. Strategies to prevent or mitigate postsurgical hypoparathyroidism are to replete vitamin D (goal $25(OH)D_3$ greater than 30 ng/mL) and also parathyroid autotransplantation, which can actually cause transient hypoparathyroidism but can be used to prevent permanent hypoparathyroidism. Parathyroid autografts typically become functional within 6 months [5].

Clinical Pearls

- Hypoparathyroidism is a condition in which the parathyroid gland does not produce enough parathyroid hormone, leading to hypocalcemia and hyperphosphatemia or high normal serum phosphorus.
- Postsurgical hypoparathyroidism results from accidental removal, devascularization, or manipulation of the parathyroid glands during thyroidectomy, parathyroidectomy, or neck surgery for head and neck cancer.
- A cutoff PTH level of 15 ng/mL at least 20 min after surgery can be used to help determine whether a patient may be discharged the same day or needs overnight observation.
- Symptoms of hypocalcemia to monitor for after surgery include paresthesias, cramping, carpopedal spasm, confusion, etc.
- Oral calcium and calcitriol and correction of hypomagnesemia or vitamin D deficiency are the treatment for hypoparathyroidism. A continuous calcium gluconate drip may be needed in addition to oral medications if the patient has acute symptoms or corrected serum calcium <7.5 mg/dL.
- Most postsurgical hypoparathyroidism is transient and resolves within 6 months.

Suggested Reading

1. Khan MI, Waguespack SG, Hu MI. Medical management of postsurgical hypoparathyroidism. Endocr Pract. 2011;17 Suppl 1, 18–25.
2. Stack BC, Jr., Bimston DN, Bodenner DL, et al. American association of clinical endocrinologists and American College of

endocrinology disease state clinical review: postoperative hypoparathyroidism – definitions and management. Endocr Pract.
2015;21(6), 674–85.

References

1. Khan MI, Waguespack SG, Hu MI. Medical management of postsurgical
   hypoparathyroidism. Endocr Pract. 2011;17 Suppl 1:18–25.
2. Noordzij JP, Lee SL, Bernet VJ, et al. Early prediction of hypocalcemia
   after thyroidectomy using parathyroid hormone: an analysis of pooled individual patient data from nine observational studies. J Am Coll Surg.
   2007;205(6):748–54.
3. Kim ES, Keating GM. Recombinant human parathyroid hormone (1-84): a
   review in hypoparathyroidism. Drugs. 2015;75(11):1293–303.
4. Puig-Domingo M, Diaz G, Nicolau J, et al. Successful treatment of vitamin
   D unresponsive hypoparathyroidism with multipulse subcutaneous infusion
   of teriparatide. Eur J Endocrinol. 2008;159(5):653–7.
5. Stack Jr BC, Bimston DN, Bodenner DL, et al. American association of clinical
   endocrinologists and American College of endocrinology disease state clinical
   review: postoperative hypoparathyroidism – definitions and management.
   Endocr Pract. 2015;21(6):674–85.

Chapter 7
Vitamin D in Patients with Hypoparathyroidism/ Hypocalcemia

Tina Constantin and Vin Tangpricha

Case Presentation

A 36-year-old female was seen in consultation at the endocrinology clinic for postsurgical hypoparathyroidism after she underwent a total thyroidectomy, 5 years ago, due to compressive symptoms from a nontoxic multi-nodular goiter. The patient has had since then considerable issues with symptomatic hypocalcemia, requiring multiple hospitalizations and emergency department visits. She cannot tolerate serum calcium levels less than 9 mg/dL (normal range, 8.9–10.3 mg/dL). Her symptoms included severe peripheral paresthesia, laryngospasm, severe dyspnea, severe tetany, and

T. Constantin, M.D. (✉)
Emory University School of Medicine,
101 Woodruff Circle NE, Atlanta, GA 30322, USA

V. Tangpricha, M.D., Ph.D.
Emory University School of Medicine, Atlanta, GA, USA
e-mail: vin.tangpricha@emory.edu

© Springer International Publishing Switzerland 2016   49
V. Tangpricha (ed.), *Vitamin D*,
DOI 10.1007/978-3-319-26176-8_7

sometimes altered mental status. She also had a cardiac event due to severely symptomatic hypocalcemia. The management has been challenging given recurrent hyperphosphatemia (due to treatment with calcitriol), with calcium and phosphorus product reaching greater than 120, with persistent symptomatic hypocalcemia.

She was initially started on 1000 mg elemental calcium (calcium carbonate) three times a day, calcitriol 1 mcg twice a day, ergocalciferol 50,000 IU weekly, and chlorthalidone and levothyroxine for the postsurgical hypoparathyroidism/hypothyroidism. Furthermore, sevelamer, a phosphate binder, was added to control severe hyperphosphatemia. At one point the phosphorus levels became severely elevated ranging between 6 and 14.4 mg/dL (normal range, 2.7–4.5 mg/dL); calcitriol and calcium carbonate were discontinued temporarily until the phosphate levels normalized. She was also started on a low phosphorus diet. She was then started on calcium acetate and was continued on sevelamer. A port was also eventually placed so that the patient could receive IV calcium gluconate as needed when she is symptomatic. She sometimes required up to 6 g of IV gluconate per day.

Diagnosis/Assessment

Patients who undergo thyroidectomy are at risk for developing postoperative hypocalcemia due to transient or permanent injury to the parathyroid glands. Therefore, the serum PTH and corrected calcium should be monitored closely after surgery. The cutoff values and the timing for testing differ between centers from published studies. Most studies state that a corrected serum calcium of less than 8.0 postoperatively indicates hypocalcemia [1–5]. The timing of the blood sampling is critical because the earlier it is tested, the lower rates of hypocalcemia will be detected; however if it is delayed, patients might be symptomatic [1].

After thyroidectomy, it is generally recommended to check serum calcium corrected for albumin and PTH 24 hours or the morning after the surgery. If the corrected serum calcium is less than 8 mg/dL, then the patient has postoperative hypocalcemia and needs to be started on oral calcium supplementation and/or calcitriol. If the patient also has symptomatic hypocalcemia, intravenous calcium may be required in addition to calcitriol [1].

A low PTH value postoperatively indicates consistent transient or permanent injury to the parathyroid gland(s). A consistently low or undetectable PTH value indicates that patients also require calcitriol in addition to oral calcium supplementation. Parathyroid function is expected to recover in at least two thirds of patients within 1 month [1]. If treatment is needed beyond that period, then permanent surgical hypoparathyroidism is more than likely. Permanent hypoparathyroidism is defined as the need for replacement therapy for at least 6 months or 1 year after thyroidectomy. Subnormal PTH concentration (<13 pg/ml) is the usual finding in these cases [1, 6].

This patient continued to have PTH <13 with low serum calcium after 5 years of her thyroidectomy. She fits the criteria for permanent hypoparathyroidism and recovery is unlikely.

She will require lifelong calcium supplementation and calcitriol.

Management

Most recommendations for managing postsurgical hypocalcemia are based on expert opinion and clinical experience. The treatment depends on the severity of hypocalcemia, the rate of decrease of serum calcium concentrations, and presence of hypocalcemic symptoms. Patients in the acute setting may be symptomatic at higher serum calcium compared to patients with chronic hypoparathyroidism. Patient with acute hypoparathyroidism may have a rapid drop in serum calcium and PTH, leading to severe symptoms. Emergent therapy is required in the setting of tetany, seizures, or markedly prolonged QT intervals on electrocardiogram. Management of severely symptomatic hypocalcemia requires intravenous administration of one 10 mL ampule of 10 % calcium gluconate (90 mg of elemental calcium per 10 mL) in 50 mL of 5 % dextrose infused over 10–20 min, followed by an continuous intravenous infusion of calcium gluconate, because the initial loading dose will only last for 2–3 h. The calcium infusion should be given slowly, in order to prevent any serious cardiac dysfunction or arrhythmias. Oral calcium and calcitriol should be started as soon as possible, to help wean off the calcium infusion [6].

For patients with milder degree of acute hypocalcemia [serum calcium corrected for albumin of 7.5–8.0 mg/dL (1.9–2.0 mmol/L) or a serum ionized calcium concentration above 3.0–3.2 mg/dL (0.8 mmol/L)] or for chronic hypocalcemia, oral calcium is the preferred treatment. The initial dose is 1500–2000 mg of elemental calcium divided into three or four doses. In chronic stable hypoparathyroidism, the dose of oral calcium is usually 1000–2000 mg of daily elemental calcium, in divided doses. Calcium carbonate is the most commonly used oral supplementation, since it is the least expensive; however there is lower absorption in older patients or those who have low gastric acidity. In those cases, calcium citrate could be used. The goal of therapy is avoid iatrogenic nephrolithiasis and to maintain serum calcium in the low-normal range [1, 6, 7].

There are several formulations of vitamin D which are used in chronic hypoparathyroidism. There is decreased renal conversion calcidiol (25-hydroxyvitamin D [25{OH}D]) to the active metabolite calcitriol (1,25-dihydroxyvitamin D [1,25(OH)2D]) in hypoparathyroidism due to the lack of PTH; therefore, calcitriol is usually required [8]. The starting dose is 0.25 mcg once or twice a day, with weekly dose adjustments to achieve a low-normal serum calcium and phosphorus level within normal limits. One caveat of therapy is that calcitriol can also increase phosphorus concentrations [6, 8].

An emerging therapy is recombinant PTH 1–84, which is available for patients who cannot maintain stable serum calcium levels with calcium and vitamin D supplementation. In small clinical trials, it has been shown to maintain calcium levels without the need for high doses of calcium and vitamin D. It is not considered as first-line therapy because of unknown long-term safety, especially its skeletal effects and the risk for osteosarcoma, and it is much more expensive than conventional therapy [6, 9–16].

PTH 1–84 is a daily subcutaneous injection via a multi-dose injection pen device. Calcitriol is usually reduced by 50 % when treatment is started. The starting dose is 50 mcg, and the dose is titrated by 25 mcg every 4 weeks to reach a serum calcium concentration in the lower half of the normal range and to eventually discontinue calcitriol. Initially, serum calcium is measured within 3–7 days of the first dose and the dose of calcium and calcitriol is adjusted accordingly. There should also be weekly monitoring of urinary and serum calcium until calcitriol is discontinued and serum calcium is stable. Once a stable dose is reached, checking levels at 3–6 months interval is acceptable. Serum 25(OH)D should be measured Vitamin D deficiency is usually corrected to a serum 25(OH)D above 30 ng/mL [6, 17].

This patient could not maintain serum calcium in the lower half of the normal range, and she was also symptomatic at these levels. She required high doses of calcium supplementation, and calcitriol dose escalation was limited by severe hyperphosphatemia and acute kidney injury. Phosphate binders were needed in this case, and calcium citrate was used instead of calcium carbonate. In this case of chronic hypoparathyroidism, patient continued to require intravenous calcium gluconate. She is considered to be a suitable candidate for parathyroid hormone replacement, given these limitations and inability to maintain serum calcium at a safe level.

Outcome

She is currently on calcium acetate 2668 mg three times a day, calcitriol 0.25 mcg twice a day, sevelamer 2700 mg three times a day, liquid calcium 1250 mg three times a day, and chlorthalidone. Recent laboratory results showed a serum phosphate of 5.3 mg/dL (normal range, 2.7–4.5 mg/dL), a serum calcium of 10.1 mg/dL (normal range, 8.9–10.3 mg/dL), and a serum parathyroid hormone (PTH) concentration of 13 pg/mL (normal range, 14–62 pg/mL). The future plan is to start the patient on recombinant parathyroid hormone therapy.

Literature Review

The most common complication after a total thyroidectomy is post-operative hypocalcemia, whether transient (>60–70 %) or permanent [18–21]. It has a great negative impact on the patient's quality of life, since it requires rigorous follow-up, laboratory testing, and sometimes lifelong medications [1]. The estimated prevalence of postoperative hypoparathyroidism is variable; however, according to a recent meta-analysis, postoperative hypocalcemia varies from 19 to 38 % and permanent hypoparathyroidism varies from 0 to 3 %. There is variable data due to significant differences in definitions, cutoff values, and under-reporting by some centers [22].

The most common cause is acute parathyroid dysfunction due to excision, damage, or parathyroid autotransplantation [1]. Hypocalcemia is usually the result of parathyroid insufficiency leading to decreased 1,25–dihyroxyvitamin D synthesis in the kidney resulting in decreased calcium intestinal absorption and also decreased bone resorption due to decreased level of PTH. Furthermore, there is an increased risk of kidney injury, basal ganglia calcifications, neuropsychiatric dysfunctions, and infections, in the setting of chronic hypoparathyroidism [12, 16]. Barczyński et al. showed that PTH <10 pg/mL at 4 h after total thyroidectomy had a positive predictive value of 90 % for developing hypocalcemia (sCa < 8 mg/dL) after 24 h [23].

Several randomized control trials showed that administration of PTH 1–34 and 1–84, whether once or twice daily, was effective in lowering oral calcium and vitamin D requirements in patients with chronic hypoparathyroidism. Recombinant human PTH might also have skeletal benefits where BMD was shown to be significantly increased and iliac crest biopsy showed increased remodeling rate in both trabecular and cortical compartments [12, 24].

Clinical Pearls and Pitfalls

- Patients who undergo thyroidectomy are at risk for developing postoperative hypocalcemia due to transient or permanent injury to the parathyroid glands.

- Patient with acute hypoparathyroidism may have a rapid drop in serum calcium and PTH, leading to severe symptoms, and emergent therapy with intravenous calcium is required.
- Permanent hypoparathyroidism is defined as the need for replacement therapy for at least 6 months or 1 year after thyroidectomy.
- The conventional therapy of chronic hypoparathyroidism is oral calcium supplementation and calcitriol.
- One caveat of therapy is that calcitriol can also increase phosphorus concentrations.
- An emerging therapy is recombinant PTH 1–84, which is available for patients who cannot maintain stable serum calcium levels with calcium and vitamin D supplementation.

Suggested Reading

1. Lorente-Poch L, et al. Defining the syndromes of parathyroid failure after total thyroidectomy. Gland Surg. 2015;4(1):82–90.
2. Ramakrishnan Y, Cocks HC. Impact of recombinant PTH on management of hypoparathyroidism: a systematic review. Eur Arch Otorhinolaryngol. 2015.
3. Bergenfelz A, et al. Complications to thyroid surgery: results as reported in a database from a multicenter audit comprising 3,660 patients. Langenbecks Arch Surg. 2008;393(5):667–73.

References

1. Lorente-Poch L, et al. Defining the syndromes of parathyroid failure after total thyroidectomy. Gland Surg. 2015;4(1):82–90.
2. Thomusch O, et al. The impact of surgical technique on postoperative hypoparathyroidism in bilateral thyroid surgery: a multivariate analysis of 5846 consecutive patients. Surgery. 2003;133(2):180–5.
3. Duclos A, et al. Influence of experience on performance of individual surgeons in thyroid surgery: prospective cross sectional multicentre study. BMJ. 2012;344:d8041.

4. Hallgrimsson P, et al. Risk factors for medically treated hypocalcemia after surgery for Graves' disease: a Swedish multicenter study of 1,157 patients. World J Surg. 2012;36(8):1933–42.

5. Bergenfelz A, et al. Complications to thyroid surgery: results as reported in a database from a multicenter audit comprising 3,660 patients. Langenbecks Arch Surg. 2008;393(5):667–73.

6. Goltzman G. Hypoparathyroidism. In: Post TW, editor. UpToDate. Waltham, MA: UpToDate; 2015.

7. Sitges-Serra A, et al. Outcome of protracted hypoparathyroidism after total thyroidectomy. Br J Surg. 2010;97(11):1687–95.

8. Shoback D. Clinical practice. Hypoparathyroidism. N Engl J Med. 2008;359(4):391–403.

9. Cusano NE, et al. Therapy of hypoparathyroidism with PTH(1–84): a prospective four-year investigation of efficacy and safety. J Clin Endocrinol Metab. 2013;98(1):137–44.

10. Mannstadt M, et al. Efficacy and safety of recombinant human parathyroid hormone (1-84) in hypoparathyroidism (REPLACE): a double-blind, placebo-controlled, randomised, phase 3 study. Lancet Diabetes Endocrinol. 2013;1(4):275–83.

11. Ramakrishnan Y, Cocks HC. Impact of recombinant PTH on management of hypoparathyroidism: a systematic review. Eur Arch Otorhinolaryngol. 2015. PMID:25567344

12. Rubin MR, et al. Therapy of hypoparathyroidism with intact parathyroid hormone. Osteoporos Int. 2010;21(11):1927–34.

13. Sikjaer T, et al. The effect of adding PTH(1-84) to conventional treatment of hypoparathyroidism: a randomized, placebo-controlled study. J Bone Miner Res. 2011;26(10):2358–70.

14. Winer KK, et al. Long-term treatment of hypoparathyroidism: a randomized controlled study comparing parathyroid hormone-(1-34) versus calcitriol and calcium. J Clin Endocrinol Metab. 2003;88(9):4214–20.

15. Winer KK, Yanovski JA, Cutler Jr GB. Synthetic human parathyroid hormone 1-34 vs. calcitriol and calcium in the treatment of hypoparathyroidism. JAMA. 1996;276(8):631–6.

16. Winer KK, et al. A randomized, cross-over trial of once-daily versus twice-daily parathyroid hormone 1-34 in treatment of hypoparathyroidism. J Clin Endocrinol Metab. 1998;83(10):3480–6.

17. https://natpara.com/prescribing-information/PDF#page=1

18. Abboud B, et al. Risk factors for postthyroidectomy hypocalcemia. J Am Coll Surg. 2002;195(4):456–61.

19. Bhattacharyya N, Fried MP. Assessment of the morbidity and complications of total thyroidectomy. Arch Otolaryngol Head Neck Surg. 2002;128(4):389–92.

20. Olson Jr JA, et al. Parathyroid autotransplantation during thyroidectomy. Results of long-term follow-up. Ann Surg. 1996;223(5):472–8. discussion 478–80.

21. Pattou F, et al. Hypocalcemia following thyroid surgery: incidence and prediction of outcome. World J Surg. 1998;22(7):718–24.
22. Edafe O, et al. Systematic review and meta-analysis of predictors of post-thyroidectomy hypocalcaemia. Br J Surg. 2014;101(4):307–20.
23. Barczynski M, Cichon S, Konturek A. Which criterion of intraoperative iPTH assay is the most accurate in prediction of true serum calcium levels after thyroid surgery? Langenbecks Arch Surg. 2007;392(6):693–8.
24. Rubin MR, et al. PTH(1-84) administration reverses abnormal bone-remodeling dynamics and structure in hypoparathyroidism. J Bone Miner Res. 2011;26(11):2727–36.

Chapter 8
Vitamin D in Disorders of Phosphorus

Malcolm D. Kearns and Vin Tangpricha

Case Presentation

A 52-year-old female presented to the clinic for evaluation of bone pain. She presented initially with rachitic bone changes at the age of 2 years and was diagnosed based on laboratory findings (low phosphorous) and a potential family history of rickets (maternal family members with short stature). She was placed on 50,000 IU of vitamin D daily and phosphate five times per day. The diagnosis of X-linked hypophosphatemic rickets (XLH) was eventually confirmed by genetic testing. The patient received medical management until she was 18 and was determined to be finished with growth. However, at age 22 the patient began

M.D. Kearns, M.D. (✉)
University of Pennsylvania,
3400 Spruce St, Philadelphia, PA 19104, USA
e-mail: malcolmdkearns@gmail.com

V. Tangpricha, M.D., Ph.D.
Emory University School of Medicine, Atlanta, GA, USA
e-mail: vin.tangpricha@emory.edu

© Springer International Publishing Switzerland 2016   59
V. Tangpricha (ed.), *Vitamin D*,
DOI 10.1007/978-3-319-26176-8_8

experiencing bone pain and was started on calcitriol 0.25 mg orally twice a day and elemental phosphorous two times a day. Despite this treatment, she developed multiple rib fractures and continued to experience intermittent bone pain. Her medications were eventually titrated to phosphorus three times a day and calcitriol 0.50 mcg twice a day. Though she was stable on this regimen for many years, over the year prior to this presentation, she experienced worsening bone pain. Recent laboratory results showed a serum phosphate of 2.2 mg/dL (normal range: 2.7–4.5 mg/dL), a serum calcium of 10.4 mg/dL (normal range: 8.9–10.3 mg/dL), and a serum parathyroid hormone (PTH) concentration of 136 pg/mL (normal range, 14–62 pg/mL).

Diagnosis/Assessment

A high clinical suspicion based on family history and laboratory abnormalities consistent with XLH are grounds to initiate testing. Genetic testing may be performed to confirm the diagnosis. In children with a potential family history of rickets, laboratory testing should be performed within the first months of life, even if the child shows no signs of the disease. Measurement of serum calcium, phosphate, alkaline phosphatase (ALP), 25-hydroxyvitamin D (25(OH)D), and 1,25 dihydroxyvitamin D (1,25(OH)$_2$D or calcitriol, the active form of vitamin D) can be helpful in determining the etiology of rickets. Patients with XLH, among other forms of inherited hypophosphatemic rickets, typically have low phosphate, normal calcium, elevated ALP, and low circulating 1,25 (OH)$_2$D [1]. Laboratory values that deviate from these tend to suggest another etiology for rickets. It is important to note that phosphate levels must be adjusted for the age of the patient, since phosphate concentrations are typically elevated early in life (5.0–7.5 mg/dL) compared to adults (2.7–4.5 mg/dL) in order to promote adequate bone mineralization and dentition. Though the pathogenesis of most forms of familial hypophosphatemic rickets is related to high levels of fibroblast growth factor (FGF)-23 [2] (discussed below), FGF-23 concentrations are highly variable and not typically used in diagnosis or useful in assessing disease severity [3]. Rather, the phosphate-regulating gene homologous to endopeptidases on the X chromosome (PHEX) gene should be tested for mutations initially [4, 5]. An inactive PHEX gene is responsible for increasing FGF-23 concentrations in XLH, which comprises 80 % of patients with hypophosphatemic rickets [6]. There are many mutations of the PHEX reported.

Patients with XLH typically develop clinical evidence of the disease as they begin weight-bearing and dental development. Common abnormalities consist of decreased linear growth, lower extremity skeletal deformities, delayed dentition, and dental abscesses, though the phenotype varies even within the same family or types of mutation [7, 8]. Early recognition of XLH is essential since therapy administered during the first year of life is most effective in preventing skeletal abnormalities and short stature [7]. Radiographic images of the wrists, ankles, and long bones are useful in diagnosing rickets and tracking treatment over time. Radiographic changes in patients with XLH are identical to patients with vitamin-D deficiency rickets, including cupping and fraying of the metaphyseal region, widening of the joint spaces, and flaring of the knee joints [8].

This patient was initially diagnosed with XLH as a child and presented at this time with an established diagnosis. Though patients with XLH may often stop treatment once they are finished with growth, this patient was continued on medical management due to ongoing skeletal symptoms associated with the disease. On this admission, however, her laboratory results include elevated PTH. This is a common complication in XLH both as a result of treatment (phosphate administration increases the PTH level and induces hyperplasia in the parathyroid glands independent of calcium and calcitriol [9]) and as a consequence of the disease (FGF-23 is believed to increase PTH concentrations itself) [10].

Management

The overall aim of treatment in patients with XLH is to promote healthy bone development through replacement of serum phosphate and $1,25(OH)_2D$, which are decreased in the presence of increased serum FGF-23 (Fig. 8.1). Initiation of this treatment prior to one year of age is associated with better outcomes [7, 11], though the results are highly variable and many children fail treatment [7, 11, 12]. Treatment is typically continued until children are finished with growth, though adults with symptoms, as with this patient, can continue treatment.

The patient in this case was initially treated as a young child with inactive vitamin D (as is typically used for vitamin D deficiency) and phosphorus. This method of management is no longer commonly used; inactive vitamin D is less effective in patients with XLH due to the downregulation of CYP27B1 (the enzyme involved in converting vitamin D to its active form $1,25(OH)_2D$) by FGF-23 and because daily high-dose vitamin D greatly increases the risk of hypercalcemia. At the time of her more recent presentation, this patient was receiving a more typical regimen of elemental phosphorus three times a day and 0.50 mcg of calcitriol twice a day. Patients with XLH receiving treatment are at risk for developing hyperparathyroidism, as was seen in this patient. Thus, she was started on cinacalcet (a calcimimetic that provides negative feedback against PTH release from the parathyroid glands) at 30 mg twice a day in addition to her phosphorus and calcitriol. Nephrocalcinosis is another major complication of treatment that should be monitored for by renal ultrasonography and by measuring the calcium/creatinine ratio in the urine (a ratio >0.25:1 indicates a greater risk for nephrocalcinosis).

Outcome

Repeated laboratory values performed 3 months after initiating cinacalcet showed her serum calcium and phosphate to normalize. However, serum ALP and PTH remained elevated and she

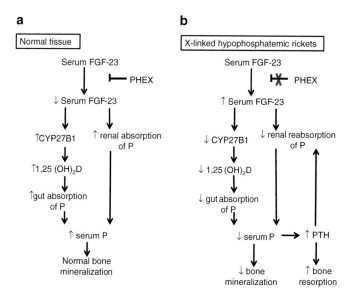

Fig. 8.1 Fibroblast growth factor (FGF)-23 regulation in normal tissue (**a**) compared to in X-linked hypophosphatemic rickets (XLH) (**b**). As shown in (**a**), serum FGF-23 is downregulated by the PHEX gene product. Decreased serum FGF-23 increases serum phosphate (P) by increasing renal absorption of P and activating CYP27B1, which increases concentrations of 1,25-dihydroxyvitamin D (1,25(OH)$_2$D) and ultimately leads to increased gut absorption of P. However, in XLH, which comprises a majority of inherited rickets, serum FGF-23 is not degraded at a normal rate due to inactive PHEX gene products. Increased FGF-23 leads to decreased serum P through decreased renal reabsorption and decreased activation of vitamin D by downregulating CYP27B1. Thus, these patients can have bone resorption and poor bone mineralization. A majority of other forms of familial hypophosphatemic rickets are also linked to defects in genes or proteins involved in downregulation or degradation of FGF-23

continued to have some lower leg pain but no fractures or other complications. Her cinacalcet dose was increased to 60 mg twice a day in an attempt to further reduce the PTH concentration and treat her continued symptoms. She was scheduled for follow-up in three months to reassess laboratory values and to perform an annual bone scan.

Literature Review

XLH is present in approximately 1 in 20,000 live births and is characterized by short stature, muscle weakness, and delayed dental development [13–15]. Though initially known as familial hypophosphatemic rickets or vitamin D-resistant rickets due to its inheritance pattern and lack of response to high-dose vitamin D, increased knowledge of the potential mutations that contribute to this phenotype has given rise to more specific subgroups of the disease. XLH, which has X-linked dominant inheritance, accounts for >80 % of patients with familial hypophosphatemic rickets [6]. The primary mutation in these patients is in the phosphate-regulating gene homologous to endopeptidases on the X chromosome (PHEX) gene [16, 17], which produces a zinc metallopeptidase [2, 18] responsible for inactivating fibroblast growth factor-23 (FGF-23) expressed in bone [19, 20]. The elevated plasma FGF-23 concentration in patients with XLH [3, 21] stimulates decreased reabsorption of phosphorous in the proximal renal tubules and decreased $1,25\text{-}(OH)_2D$ activation. These effects and the resulting hypophosphatemia contribute to the defective bone mineralization and dental abnormalities characteristic of XLH.

Increased FGF-23 concentration also contributes to the other 20 % of hypophosphatemic rickets syndromes, though through different mechanisms. For example, loss of dentin matrix acid phosphoprotein-1 (DMP-1), which forms a complex with PHEX in bone and is also involved in downregulating FGF-23 concentration, leads to an autosomal recessive form of hypophosphatemic rickets [22, 23]. Defects in ectonucleotide pyrophosphatase/phosphodiesterase 1 (ENPP1) cause a second form of autosomal recessive rickets [24] and rarely mutation on FGF-23 itself that impairs the proteolytic inactivation of FGF-23 causes an autosomal dominant form of the disease [25, 26]. Though all of these forms of hypophosphatemic rickets are related to an elevated FGF-23 concentration and significantly elevated FGF-23 concentrations (approximately 30 pg/mL and greater) are considered causative of hypophosphatemia [3, 21], the concentration of this protein is variable and poorly correlated to disease progression or clinical characteristics [3]. Thus, FGF-23 concentration is not typically involved in diagnosis of XLH. More importantly, low FGF-23 in the setting of hypophosphatemia suggests an alternative diagnosis from XLH.

Although bone disease is the most common clinical manifestation of XLH, various health complications occur secondary to dysregulation of calcium and phosphate, including hypercalcemia, nephrocalcinosis, hypertension, and hyperparathyroidism. Hypercalcemia is a primary risk of treatment with activated vitamin D (though less common than with treatment with inactive vitamin D). Though asymptomatic early in its course, hypercalcemia can lead to calcification throughout the body, such as nephrocalcinosis. Phosphate administration can also increase the risk of nephrocalcinosis, with calcium-phosphate stones forming when phosphorus becomes concentrated in the loop of Henle [2]. Maintaining a phosphate dose <60 mg/kg of body weight minimizes this risk [27]. Patients are also at risk for developing secondary hyperparathyroidism both before treatment (due to FGF-23 stimulation of the parathyroid glands [10]) and as a result of phosphate administration [9].

Beyond standard treatments of XLH with phosphorus and calcitriol, several investigative therapies exist. Evidence suggests that calcitonin stimulates $1,25(OH)_2D$ in XLH and healthy controls [28] and reduces circulating levels of FGF-23 [29]. Some studies suggest that growth hormone (GH) administration may improve growth velocity [30, 31] and increase renal phosphate reabsorption and CYP27B1 activity [32]. In addition, anti-FGF-23 neutralizing antibodies may also be beneficial in future treatments based on some evidence in mouse models [33, 34].

Clinical Pearls/Pitfalls

- XLH accounts for 80 % of inherited hypophosphatemic rickets. This and other forms of hypophosphatemic rickets are related to elevated serum FGF-23, which causes hypophosphatemia and decreased $1,25(OH)_2D$ activation.
- The diagnosis of XLH and involves a high suspicion of the disease by family history followed by laboratory abnormalities

(low phosphate, normal calcium, high ALP). Genetic testing is available though results are poorly correlated with clinical findings or disease progression.

- Early recognition and treatment of XLH is essential since children treated after age 1 experience worse linear growth compared to children treated at earlier ages.
- Standard treatment of XLH involves elemental phosphorus and $1,25(OH)_2D$ administration, though response to this treatment is variable.
- Secondary hyperparathyroidism frequently occurs in these patients either as a result of the disease or as an effect of treatment.
- Genetic counselling following diagnosis of XLH can aid patients and their families in appreciating the implications of the diagnosis.

Suggested Reading

1. Lee JY, Imel EA. The changing face of hypophosphatemic disorders in the FGF-23 era. Pediatr Endocrinol Rev. 2013;10 Suppl 2:367–79.
2. Baroncelli GI, Toschi B, Bertelloni S. Hypophosphatemic rickets. Curr Opin Endocrinol Diabetes Obes. 2012;19(6):460–7.

References

1. Carpenter TO. The expanding family of hypophosphatemic syndromes. J Bone Miner Metab. 2012;30(1):1–9.
2. Prie D, Friedlander G. Genetic disorders of renal phosphate transport. N Engl J Med. 2010;362(25):2399–409.
3. Igaki JM, Yamada M, Yamazaki Y, Koto S, Izawa M, Ariyasu D, et al. High iFGF23 level despite hypophosphatemia is one of the clinical indicators to make diagnosis of XLH. Endocr J. 2011;58(8):647–55.
4. Kinoshita Y, Saito T, Shimizu Y, Hori M, Taguchi M, Igarashi T, et al. Mutational analysis of patients with FGF23-related hypophosphatemic rickets. Eur J Endocrinol. 2012;167(2):165–72.

5. Beck-Nielsen SS, Brixen K, Gram J, Brusgaard K. Mutational analysis of PHEX, FGF23, DMP1, SLC34A3 and CLCN5 in patients with hypophosphatemic rickets. J Hum Genet. 2012;57(7):453–8.

6. Nielsen LH, Rahbek ET, Beck-Nielsen SS, Christesen HT. Treatment of hypophosphataemic rickets in children remains a challenge. Dan Med J. 2014;61(7):A4874.

7. Quinlan C, Guegan K, Offiah A, Neill RO, Hiorns MP, Ellard S, et al. Growth in PHEX-associated X-linked hypophosphatemic rickets: the importance of early treatment. Pediatr Nephrol. 2012;27(4):581–8.

8. Econs MJ, Feussner JR, Samsa GP, Effman EL, Vogler JB, Martinez S, et al. X-linked hypophosphatemic rickets without "rickets". Skelet Radiol. 1991;20(2):109–14.

9. Slatopolsky E, Finch J, Denda M, Ritter C, Zhong M, Dusso A, et al. Phosphorus restriction prevents parathyroid gland growth. High phosphorus directly stimulates PTH secretion in vitro. J Clin Invest. 1996;97(11):2534–40.

10. Hasegawa H, Nagano N, Urakawa I, Yamazaki Y, Iijima K, Fujita T, et al. Direct evidence for a causative role of FGF23 in the abnormal renal phosphate handling and vitamin D metabolism in rats with early-stage chronic kidney disease. Kidney Int. 2010;78(10):975–80.

11. Makitie O, Doria A, Kooh SW, Cole WG, Daneman A, Sochett E. Early treatment improves growth and biochemical and radiographic outcome in X-linked hypophosphatemic rickets. J Clin Endocrinol Metab. 2003;88(8):3591–7.

12. Petersen DJ, Boniface AM, Schranck FW, Rupich RC, Whyte MP. X-linked hypophosphatemic rickets: a study (with literature review) of linear growth response to calcitriol and phosphate therapy. J Bone Miner Res. 1992;7(6):583–97.

13. Santos F, Fuente R, Mejia N, Mantecon L, Gil-Pena H, Ordonez FA. Hypophosphatemia and growth. Pediatr Nephrol. 2013;28(4):595–603.

14. Opsahl Vital S, Gaucher C, Bardet C, Rowe PS, George A, Linglart A, et al. Tooth dentin defects reflect genetic disorders affecting bone mineralization. Bone. 2012;50(4):989–97.

15. Veilleux LN, Cheung M, Ben Amor M, Rauch F. Abnormalities in muscle density and muscle function in hypophosphatemic rickets. J Clin Endocrinol Metab. 2012;97(8):E1492–8.

16. Francis F, Strom TM, Hennig S, Boddrich A, Lorenz B, Brandau O, et al. Genomic organization of the human PEX gene mutated in X-linked dominant hypophosphatemic rickets. Genome Res. 1997;7(6):573–85.

17. Rowe PS. The role of the PHEX gene (PEX) in families with X-linked hypophosphataemic rickets. Curr Opin Nephrol Hypertens. 1998; 7(4):367–76.

18. Cho HY, Lee BH, Kang JH, Ha IS, Cheong HI, Choi Y. A clinical and molecular genetic study of hypophosphatemic rickets in children. Pediatr Res. 2005;58(2):329–33.

19. Burckhardt MA, Schifferli A, Krieg AH, Baumhoer D, Szinnai G, Rudin C. Tumor-associated FGF-23-induced hypophosphatemic rickets in children: a case report and review of the literature. Pediatr Nephrol. 2015;30(1):179–82.

20. Zou M, Bulus D, Al-Rijjal RA, Andiran N, BinEssa H, Kattan WE, et al. Hypophosphatemic rickets caused by a novel splice donor site mutation and activation of two cryptic splice donor sites in the PHEX gene. J Pediatr Endocrinol Metab. 2015;28(1–2):211–6.

21. Endo I, Fukumoto S, Ozono K, Namba N, Tanaka H, Inoue D, et al. Clinical usefulness of measurement of fibroblast growth factor 23 (FGF23) in hypophosphatemic patients: proposal of diagnostic criteria using FGF23 measurement. Bone. 2008;42(6):1235–9.

22. Feng JQ, Ward LM, Liu S, Lu Y, Xie Y, Yuan B, et al. Loss of DMP1 causes rickets and osteomalacia and identifies a role for osteocytes in mineral metabolism. Nat Genet. 2006;38(11):1310–5.

23. Lorenz-Depiereux B, Bastepe M, Benet-Pages A, Amyere M, Wagenstaller J, Muller-Barth U, et al. DMP1 mutations in autosomal recessive hypophosphatemia implicate a bone matrix protein in the regulation of phosphate homeostasis. Nat Genet. 2006;38(11):1248–50.

24. Saito T, Shimizu Y, Hori M, Taguchi M, Igarashi T, Fukumoto S, et al. A patient with hypophosphatemic rickets and ossification of posterior longitudinal ligament caused by a novel homozygous mutation in ENPP1 gene. Bone. 2011;49(4):913–6.

25. Alon US. Clinical practice. Fibroblast growth factor (FGF)23: a new hormone. Eur J Pediatr. 2011;170(5):545–54.

26. Gattineni J, Baum M. Genetic disorders of phosphate regulation. Pediatr Nephrol. 2012;27(9):1477–87.

27. Verge CF, Lam A, Simpson JM, Cowell CT, Howard NJ, Silink M. Effects of therapy in X-linked hypophosphatemic rickets. N Engl J Med. 1991;325(26):1843–8.

28. Econs MJ, Lobaugh B, Drezner MK. Normal calcitonin stimulation of serum calcitriol in patients with X-linked hypophosphatemic rickets. J Clin Endocrinol Metab. 1992;75(2):408–11.

29. Liu ES, Carpenter TO, Gundberg CM, Simpson CA, Insogna KL. Calcitonin administration in X-linked hypophosphatemia. N Engl J Med. 2011;364(17):1678–80.

30. Seikaly MG, Brown R, Baum M. The effect of recombinant human growth hormone in children with X-linked hypophosphatemia. Pediatrics. 1997;100(5):879–84.

31. Baroncelli GI, Bertelloni S, Ceccarelli C, Saggese G. Effect of growth hormone treatment on final height, phosphate metabolism, and bone mineral density in children with X-linked hypophosphatemic rickets. J Pediatr. 2001;138(2):236–43.

32. Feld S, Hirschberg R. Growth hormone, the insulin-like growth factor system, and the kidney. Endocr Rev. 1996;17(5):423–80.

33. Aono Y, Hasegawa H, Yamazaki Y, Shimada T, Fujita T, Yamashita T, et al. Anti-FGF-23 neutralizing antibodies ameliorate muscle weakness and decreased spontaneous movement of Hyp mice. J Bone Miner Res. 2011;26(4):803–10.
34. Shimada T, Fukumoto S. FGF23 as a novel therapeutic target. Adv Exp Med Biol. 2012;728:158–70.

Chapter 9
Vitamin D in Disorders of Vitamin D Action: Vitamin D-Dependent Rickets Type I

Oranan Siwamogsatham and Vin Tangpricha

Case Presentation

A 2-year-old previously healthy Thai girl presented with a 9-month history of regression of gross motor milestones and failure to thrive. She had been pulling to stand and walking at the age of 9 and 12 months, respectively. At 15 months of age, she lost the ability to stand holding on, and by the time of presentation, her gross motor regressed to only being able to sit without support. Her personal social, receptive language, and expressive language were well preserved. She was the only child born to non-consanguineous parents, with no family history of familial hereditary disease or metabolic

O. Siwamogsatham, M.D. (✉)
Samitivej Children's Hospital, Bangkok Hospital Group,
488 Srinakarin Road, Suanluang, Bangkok 10250, Thailand
e-mail: oranan.w@gmail.com

V. Tangpricha, M.D., Ph.D.
Emory University School of Medicine, Atlanta, GA, USA
e-mail: vin.tangpricha@emory.edu

© Springer International Publishing Switzerland 2016
V. Tangpricha (ed.), *Vitamin D*,
DOI 10.1007/978-3-319-26176-8_9

bone disease. She consumed 28 oz of milk daily. She was adequately exposed to sunlight. On the examination, her weight was 8.5 kg (−2.6 SDS), her length was 74 cm (−3.8 SDS), and upper/lower segment ratio was 1.5:1. Her anterior fontanelle was large. Rachitic rosary, genu varum, and widening of wrists and ankles were observed. Otherwise the remainder of the exam was normal.

Diagnosis/Assessment

A skeletal survey revealed widened uncalcified epiphyses, fraying, flaring, and cupping of metaphyses and osteopenia. Initial biochemical finding showed low serum calcium (5.3 mg/dL), slightly low serum phosphorus for age (3.8 mg/dL), high serum alkaline phosphatase (1409 U/L), and elevated parathyroid hormone (PTH) level (91.6 pg/mL). Serum 25-hydroxyvitamin D (25(OH)D) was normal at 38 ng/mL. Urine calcium/Cr was low (0.025 mg/mg). Renal function and serum electrolytes were normal. The history of developmental regression of motor skills and disproportionate short stature coupled with radiological finding of rickets and laboratory findings that show low serum calcium, slightly low serum phosphorus, high serum alkaline phosphatase, and elevated PTH level was consistent with the diagnosis of nutritional rickets. The differential diagnosis in addition to nutritional rickets included a defect of vitamin D metabolism. From the history, she consumed adequate amount of milk and her vitamin D status was normal by her serum 25(OH)D concentration.

Excluding nutritional rickets as a cause, the most likely diagnosis was a vitamin D metabolism defect. There are two major types of vitamin D metabolism defects including vitamin D-dependent rickets type I (VDDR I) caused by a mutation in *CYP27B1* gene that impairs the conversion of 25(OH)D to 1,25-dihydroxyvitamin D ($1,25(OH)_2D$) and vitamin D-dependent rickets type II (VDDR II) or vitamin D-resistant rickets, caused by the mutation of vitamin D receptor. The *CYP27B1* gene mutation analysis in this patient revealed missense mutation (R453H) and insertion (p.F443fsX466) on exon 8, which confirms the diagnosis of VDDR I. Both parents were heterogeneous carrier of the mutation.

Management

The initial management of VDDR I with hypocalcemia includes aggressive calcium and calcitriol supplementation. In this patient, 10 % calcium gluconate (1 mL/kg) was given intravenously every 6 h along with oral calcitriol 1.5 mcg/day and oral calcium 1600 mg of elemental calcium in divided doses per day in attempts to raise the serum calcium into the normal range. One week after treatment, her serum calcium remained low (5.2 mg/dL). Oral calcitriol was increased to 3 mcg and oral calcium was increased to 2500 mg per day in order to normalize serum calcium. In spite of continually increasing doses of calcitriol and oral and intravenous calcium, her serum calcium still remained persistently low (5.8 mg/dL) after 2 weeks of treatment. The calcitriol dose was then titrated up to 5.25 mcg a day to maintain serum calcium in a more acceptable level of 7 mg/dL. Intravenous calcium was then discontinued at day 19 of treatment. After discontinuation of intravenous calcium, her serum calcium remained normal at 9 mg/dL. Soon after the discontinuation of the intravenous calcium, the oral calcitriol dose was decreased to 0.25 mcg daily and her calcium supplementation decreased to 250 mg of elemental calcium daily.

Outcome

Three months after treatment, she could stand by holding on and walk independently. Her laboratory tests revealed normal serum calcium (10.4 mg/dL), normal serum phosphorus (4.9 mg/dL), slightly elevated serum alkaline phosphatase (347 U/L), and normal PTH level (29.8 pg/mL). Her serum alkaline phosphatase level returned to normal (181 U/L) 6 months after treatment. At a follow-up visit at the age of 4 years, she continued taking calcitriol 0.25 mcg and calcium 250 mg of elemental calcium a day. She had normal growth (body weight and height at 50th centile) and normal development. Her serum calcium, phosphorus, alkaline phosphatase, and PTH levels remained normal.

Literature Review

Rickets is a disease of bone in children characterized by impaired mineralization of the bone matrix. During endochondral bone formation in children, the bone matrix is laid down and subsequently mineralized. When endochondral osteoid is not fully mineralized, the ends of the long bone, particularly those that are weight bearing, deform and rickets ensues. Clinically, rickets is manifested by delayed closure of fontanelles, frontal bossing, delayed tooth eruption with poor enamel, genu varum or genu valgum, flaring of the metaphyses of long bone, and tibial or femoral torsion. Radiographically, rickets is characterized by cupping, splaying, and fraying of metaphyses of long bone and demineralization. Vitamin D is the principal hormone required for normal bone mineralization. Dietary vitamin D deficiency and genetic disorders of vitamin D biosynthesis can cause rickets. Hypophosphatemia due to renal phosphate wasting, renal tubular acidosis, and hypophosphatasia also can cause rickets [1, 2] as well as inadequate dietary intake of calcium or phosphorus.

Vitamin D is an inactive hormone precursor, requiring two hydroxylation steps, first in the liver to 25(OH)D by 25-hydroxylase enzyme and then in the kidney to $1,25(OH)_2D$ by 1α-hydroxylase enzyme. The hormonal form of vitamin D, $1,25(OH)_2D$, specifically binds to vitamin D receptor to mediate the actions of the hormone. Vitamin D-dependent rickets type 1 results when the 1α-hydroxylase enzyme (*CYP27B1*) is mutated and rendered defective. Vitamin D-dependent rickets type II or vitamin D-resistant rickets develops when there is a mutation of the vitamin D receptor [3–5].

VDDR I, also known as pseudovitamin D deficiency rickets, is an autosomal recessive disorder. The clinical course and presentation are similar to nutritional vitamin D deficiency rickets. Affected children appear normal at birth, but develop typical features of rickets including bone deformities, growth retardation, muscle weakness, and/or seizure within the first to second years of life. Classical biochemical findings are hypocalcemia, hypophosphatemia, and elevated serum level of PTH. The diagnosis of VDDR I is established by finding normal serum concentrations of 25(OH)D but extremely low or undetectable 1,25-dihydroxyvitamin D concentration. The diagnosis is confirmed by identification of the mutation in *CYP27B1*. The clinical, biochemical, and radiographic manifestation of VDDR I resolves following treatment with physiologic amounts of calcitriol as well as providing sufficient amounts of calcium and phosphorus to properly mineralize the skeleton [6, 7].

Clinical Pearls/Pitfalls

- Rickets in children that occurs with adequate calcium and vitamin D nutrition should prompt investigation for other genetic forms of rickets, including those that impact vitamin D metabolism.
- Correction of vitamin D-dependent rickets type I or II requires treatment with calcium and the active form of vitamin D, calcitriol.
- Vitamin D-dependent rickets type I occurs from mutations of the 1-alpha-hydroxylase, whereas vitamin D-dependent rickets type II occurs from mutations of the vitamin D receptor.

Acknowledgments We thank Preamrudee Poomthavorn, M.D., and Pat Mahachokletwattana, M.D., from the Division of Endocrinology and Metabolism, Department of Pediatrics, Ramathibodi Hospital, Mahidol University, Bangkok, Thailand, for providing clinical data on this patient.

References

1. Root AW, Diamond FB. Disorder of mineral homeostasis in newborn, infant, child and adolescent. In: Sperling MA, editor. Pediatric endocrinology. 3rd ed. Philadephia: Saunders; 2008. p. 686–769.
2. Miller WL, Portale AA. Genetic causes of rickets. Curr Opin Pediatr. 1999;11(4):333–9.
3. Kato S, Yoshizazawa T, Kitanaka S, Murayama A, Takeyama K. Molecular genetics of vitamin D-dependent hereditary rickets. Horm Res. 2002; 57(3–4):73–8.
4. Malloy PJ, Feldman D. Genetic disorders and defects in vitamin D action. Endocrinol Metab Clin N Am. 2010;39(2):333–46.

5. Kitanaka S, Takeyama K, Murayama A, Kato S. The molecular basis of vitamin D-dependent rickets type I. Endocr J. 2001;48(4):427–32.
6. Miller WL, Portale AA. Genetics of vitamin D biosynthesis and its disorders. Best Pract Res Clin Endocrinol Metab. 2001;15(1):95–109.
7. Durmaz E, Zou M, Al-Rijjal RA, Bircan I, Akcurin S, Meyer B, Shi Y. Clinical and genetic analysis of patients with vitamin D-dependent rickets type 1A. Clin Endocrinol. 2012;77(3):363–9.

Chapter 10
Vitamin D Deficiency in Chronic Kidney Disease

Malcolm D. Kearns and Vin Tangpricha

Case Presentation

A 64-year-old African American female with years of stable chronic kidney disease (CKD) secondary to hypertension and diabetes (baseline creatinine 2.0 mg/dL) presented to clinic for evaluation of hypercalcemia. Ten years prior to this presentation, the patient had a parathyroid surgery due to hyperparathyroidism. Several years following the surgery, she began experiencing dizzy spells associated with mild hypercalcemia and elevated intact parathyroid hormone (iPTH) levels. This worsened dramatically in the year prior to this presentation; the patient's iPTH was measured as high as 523 pg/mL (laboratory range, 10–65 pg/mL), with a serum calcium of 11.8 mg/dL (laboratory range, 8.9–10.3 mg/dL), low serum

M.D. Kearns, M.D. (✉)
University of Pennsylvania, 3400 Spruce St,
Philadelphia, PA 19104, USA
e-mail: malcolmdkearns@gmail.com

V. Tangpricha, M.D., Ph.D.
Emory University School of Medicine, Atlanta, GA, USA
e-mail: vin.tangpricha@emory.edu

© Springer International Publishing Switzerland 2016
V. Tangpricha (ed.), *Vitamin D*,
DOI 10.1007/978-3-319-26176-8_10

25-hydroxyvitamin D (25(OH)D), and normal serum 1,25-dihy-droxyvitamin D (1,25(OH)$_2$D). She had no symptoms associated with her hypercalcemia aside from dizziness. Several medications (nasal calcitonin, bisphosphonates) were unsuccessful in controlling her calcium. An oral form of calcitriol was tried to lower her PTH but worsened her hypercalcemia. Her estimated glomerular filtration rate (eGFR) was calculated to be <60 mL/min/1.73 m^2 at presentation.

Diagnosis/Assessment

In the setting of CKD, the combination of low vitamin D levels (due to decreased activation and reabsorption in the kidney), elevated phosphorus (due to decreased renal excretion), and hypocalcemia (due to poor intestinal absorption) can lead to hypersecretion of PTH from the parathyroid glands, or secondary hyperparathyroidism. Secondary hyperparathyroidism likely prompted the initial parathyroid gland surgery in this patient. However, years following surgery, this patient once again began to experience hyperparathyroidism, though this time it was in the setting of hypercalcemia. Patients with secondary hyperparathyroidism typically have normal calcium concentrations since the parathyroid glands remain responsive to negative feedback from increasing serum calcium concentrations.

Hypercalcemia in the setting of extremely elevated PTH suggests tertiary hyperparathyroidism, or the autonomous release of PTH from the parathyroid glands, which often occurs in patients who have experienced secondary hyperparathyroidism for years. The chronic over-secretion of PTH can contribute to hyperplasia of the parathyroid tissue and ultimately form monoclonal nodules (known as nodular hyperplasia) with altered surface receptors that make these cells unresponsive to normal regulatory feedback. In the long term, the altered parathyroid glands can often autonomously secrete PTH. While a parathyroidectomy is often a definitive treatment for either secondary or tertiary hyperparathyroidism, the rate of recurrent hyperparathyroidism following surgery is between 5 and 20 % [1].

Management

Although surgical re-exploration would be one option for treatment in this patient, medical management alone can often provide adequate PTH reduction. The initial treatment for patients with secondary/tertiary hyperparathyroidism often involves correction of vitamin D status, normalizing phosphate concentrations, and administration of activated vitamin D (used cautiously in patients with borderline or high calcium concentrations). Since this patient presented with hypercalcemia and after failing several of these therapies, she was started on cinacalcet at 20 mg daily. Cinacalcet is a calcimimetic, meaning it mimics the action of calcium in activating the calcium-sensing receptor (CaSR) in the parathyroid glands and thus allows for smaller increases in blood calcium to trigger negative feedback to decrease PTH release. Treatment with cinacalcet is also less likely to cause hypercalcemia, as occurred with calcitriol in this patient.

The measurable goals of treatment are outlined in the National Kidney Foundation Kidney Disease Outcomes Quality Initiative (NKF KDOQI) guidelines. For this patient, who has either stage 3 (GFR 30–59 mL/min/1.73 m^2) or stage 4 (GFR 15–29 mL/min/1.73 m^2) CKD, iPTH should be between 35 and 70 pg/mL or 70–110 pg/mL, respectively [2]. Along with PTH concentration, it is also important to evaluate serum calcium, serum phosphorus, and calcium phosphorus product (Ca×P), which are all linked to increased mortality in CKD patients when elevated [3, 4]. Performing regular bone mineral density (BMD) screening is also important in order to evaluate for osteopenia. In addition to cinacalcet, this patient received vitamin D to replete her vitamin D deficiency.

Outcome

One month following her presentation, the patient experienced a significant decrease in calcium (to 10.9 mg/dL) and iPTH (to 189 pg/mL). In an attempt to further decrease her PTH and calcium, her dose of cinacalcet was gradually increased. In spite of this, her iPTH continued to fluctuate between 150 and 300 pg/mL and her calcium remained between 10.2 and 10.9 mg/dL. She eventually reached the KDOQI goals in terms of calcium and PTH levels on a dose of 90 mg of cinacalcet orally twice daily. At this time she was vitamin D sufficient (maintained with a monthly 50,000 IU dose of vitamin D$_2$) and her BMD scan was normal aside from osteopenia in one hip (T-score −1.4).

However, after two years of stable laboratory values on the above regimen, her iPTH rose to 265 pg/mL. Her serum calcium, phosphorus, and 25(OH)D concentrations were within normal limits and her creatinine was stable at that time. Paricalcitol (1 mcg per day), an oral calcitriol analogue, was then added to her medication regimen. Paricalcitol was added cautiously since she had experienced hypercalcemia on similar agents in the past. Ultimately, the patient was able to achieve and maintain PTH levels at goal with normal calcium and vitamin D status and stable BMD on cinacalcet (90 mg twice daily) and paricalcitol (1 mcg daily). After several years, the patient's kidney function gradually worsened and she was evaluated for kidney transplant.

Literature Review

Secondary hyperparathyroidism is a common abnormality CKD and is related to numerous factors that can occur as the GFR falls below 60 mL/min/1.73 m^2 [3, 5]. For example, vitamin D deficiency can lead to decreased calcium absorption in the gut and thus decreased activation of the CaSR in the parathyroid gland and increased PTH secretion. PTH in turn up-regulates the 1-alpha-hydroxylation of 25(OH)D in the kidney in order to increase circulating levels of 1,25(OH)$_2$D and thus normalize calcium through increased intestinal absorption. However, renal damage, and often low 25(OH)D due to reduced reabsorption in the kidney, makes CKD patients unable to increase 1,25(OH)$_2$D concentrations sufficiently to down-regulate the PTH gene [6, 7]. Furthermore, FGF-23 is frequently elevated in patients with CKD which can further inhibit the 1-alpha-hydroxylation of 25(OH)D in the kidney. Another cause of increased PTH secretion in patients with CKD is due to decreased phosphorus excretion in the kidney. Since PTH release can be stimulated by elevated blood phosphorus in order to increase phosphorus excretion in the kidney, decreased phosphorus excretion can create a cycle of increased phosphorus and thus increased PTH.

The stimuli of hypocalcemia, $1,25(OH)_2D$ deficiency, and phosphorus retention can induce cell proliferation in the parathyroid glands and can cause parathyroid hyperplasia [8, 9]. As CKD progresses and parathyroid hyperplasia worsens, some parathyroid gland cells can escape from the cell cycle and form nodules, a process known as nodular hyperplasia [8]. These changes alter the characteristics of the cells in the parathyroid gland, for example, down-regulating the vitamin D receptor (VDR) [10] and CaSR [11] in the parathyroid glands, ultimately making the them less responsive to typical negative feedback mechanisms [8, 12]. In the long term, the altered parathyroid glands can often autonomously secrete PTH, which is known as tertiary hyperparathyroidism.

Ultimately, this process can have negative health consequences for individuals with CKD; increased PTH, phosphorus, and $Ca \times P$ are associated with mortality due to cardiac complications [3, 4] and concentrations of bone turnover markers correlate with both PTH levels and GFR [13]. Thus, serial measurements of PTH, calcium, and phosphorus are important as renal function decreases. Due to high intraindividual variation in PTH concentrations, multiple measurements of PTH concentration can be necessary to accurately assess an individual's PTH concentration [14]. As described above, the KDOQI guidelines suggest goal PTH, calcium, phosphorus, $Ca \times P$, and $25(OH)D$ concentrations for patients with CKD depending on their stage [2].

In the past, parathyroidectomy has been a definitive cure for many patients with hyperparathyroidism. However, current medical therapies can delay or entirely prevent the need for surgery in many patients. For example, restriction of dietary phosphorus (or potentially the use of oral phosphorus binders in patients with more severe hyperphosphatemia) can suppress PTH hypersecretion independent of calcium or calcitriol [15, 16]. Decreased calcitriol production also contributes to secondary hyperparathyroidism [17]; the administration of calcitriol decreases PTH gene expression in mouse models [18]. However, although activated forms of vitamin D are effective and are the primary therapy for prevention and treatment of secondary hyperparathyroidism in dialysis patients

[19, 20], these medications can lead to hypercalcemia and hyper-phosphatemia through increased gut absorption of calcium and phosphorus. For example, paricalcitol, as was given to this patient, caused as many as 60 % of patients to have elevations in calcium or $Ca \times P$ levels [21]. Calcimimetics, such as cinacalcet, increase extracellular calcium sensitivity of the CaSR within 1–2 h of administration [22, 23] and can improve the ability of conventional treatment strategies to reach treatment goals [24, 25] with less elevation of calcium and phosphorus [24, 26]. While calcimimetics can be used on their own, one study [27] showed a significantly greater proportion of subjects receiving cinacalcet and calcitriol to achieve PTH <300 pg/mL along with less hypercalcemia compared to participants who used calcitriol alone to treat secondary hyper-parathyroidism in CKD.

Some studies suggest that imaging can be used to predict the responsiveness of a patient to treatment. For example, parathyroid glands measured on ultrasound to be larger than 0.5 cm^3 or 1 cm in diameter [28] or glands heavier than 0.5 g [26] are more likely to be refractory to calcitriol therapy, likely due to increased nodular hyperplasia. Thus, patients with larger parathyroid glands who do not respond to short courses of treatment should likely receive surgical therapy or treatment by direct injection with ethanol or calcitriol [29, 30].

Clinical Pearls/Pitfalls

- Hyperparathyroidism in patients with CKD is very common. Though a majority of cases are due to secondary hyperparathyroidism, a clinician must be careful to assess for autonomy or other causes when laboratory values are not as expected (e.g., hypercalcemia).
- Current medical therapy can allow for delay of surgery in many patients.
- In patients with tertiary hyperparathyroidism, activated vitamin D, such as paricalcitol, should be used secondarily to calcimimetics since they can exacerbate hypercalcemia in a patient prone to hypercalcemia. Though effective on their own, calcimimetics can both increase the efficacy of these medications and reduce

the risk of hypercalcemia and hyperphosphatemia when used along with calcitriol.

* Regular BMD screening is important to assess the possibility for metabolic bone disease in patients with hyperparathyroidism.
* Imaging of parathyroid hormone tissue is not essential in the medical management of hyperparathyroidism, though the assessment of the size of parathyroid glands using ultrasound can help to predict the responsiveness of the patient to treatment.

Suggested Reading

1. Fukagawa M, Nakanishi S, Kazama JJ. Basic and clinical aspects of parathyroid hyperplasia in chronic kidney disease. Kidney Int Suppl. 2006(102):S3–7.
2. Joy MS, Kshirsagar AV, Franceschini N. Calcimimetics and the treatment of primary and secondary hyperparathyroidism. Ann Pharmacother. 2004;38(11):1871–80.
3. Low TH, Clark J, Gao K, Eris J, Shannon K, O'Brien C. Outcome of parathyroidectomy for patients with renal disease and hyperparathyroidism: predictors for recurrent hyperparathyroidism. ANZ J Surg. 2009;79(5):378–82.

References

1. Low TH, Clark J, Gao K, Eris J, Shannon K, O'Brien C. Outcome of parathyroidectomy for patients with renal disease and hyperparathyroidism: predictors for recurrent hyperparathyroidism. ANZ J Surg. 2009; 79(5):378–82.
2. Foundation NK. K/DOQI clinical practice guidelines for bone metabolism and disease in chronic kidney disease. Am J Kidney Dis. 2003;42 Suppl 3:S1–201.
3. Llach F, Yudd M. Pathogenic, clinical, and therapeutic aspects of secondary hyperparathyroidism in chronic renal failure. Am J Kidney Dis. 1998;32(2 Suppl 2):S3–12.
4. Raggi P, Boulay A, Chasan-Taber S, Amin N, Dillon M, Burke SK, et al. Cardiac calcification in adult hemodialysis patients. A link between end-stage renal disease and cardiovascular disease? J Am Coll Cardiol. 2002;39(4):695–701.

5. Coresh J, Astor BC, Greene T, Eknoyan G, Levey AS. Prevalence of chronic kidney disease and decreased kidney function in the adult US population: third national health and nutrition examination survey. Am J Kidney Dis. 2003;41(1):1–12.

6. DeLuca HF, Zierold C. Mechanisms and functions of vitamin D. Nutr Rev. 1998;56(2 Pt 2):S4–10. discussion S54–75.

7. Brenza HL, Kimmel-Jehan C, Jehan F, Shinki T, Wakino S, Anazawa H, et al. Parathyroid hormone activation of the 25-hydroxyvitamin D3-1alpha-hydroxylase gene promoter. Proc Natl Acad Sci U S A. 1998;95(4):1387–91.

8. Drueke TB. Cell biology of parathyroid gland hyperplasia in chronic renal failure. J Am Soc Nephrol. 2000;11(6):1141–52.

9. Naveh-Many T, Rahamimov R, Livni N, Silver J. Parathyroid cell proliferation in normal and chronic renal failure rats. The effects of calcium, phosphate, and vitamin D. J Clin Invest. 1995;96(4):1786–93.

10. Fukuda N, Tanaka H, Tominaga Y, Fukagawa M, Kurokawa K, Seino Y. Decreased 1,25-dihydroxyvitamin D3 receptor density is associated with a more severe form of parathyroid hyperplasia in chronic uremic patients. J Clin Invest. 1993;92(3):1436–43.

11. Gogusev J, Duchambon P, Hory B, Giovannini M, Goureau Y, Sarfati E, et al. Depressed expression of calcium receptor in parathyroid gland tissue of patients with hyperparathyroidism. Kidney Int. 1997;51(1):328–36.

12. Fukagawa M, Nakanishi S, Kazama JJ. Basic and clinical aspects of parathyroid hyperplasia in chronic kidney disease. Kidney Int Suppl. 2006; 102:S3–7.

13. Rix M, Andreassen H, Eskildsen P, Langdahl B, Olgaard K. Bone mineral density and biochemical markers of bone turnover in patients with predialysis chronic renal failure. Kidney Int. 1999;56(3):1084–93.

14. Gardham C, Stevens PE, Delaney MP, LeRoux M, Coleman A, Lamb EJ. Variability of parathyroid hormone and other markers of bone mineral metabolism in patients receiving hemodialysis. Clin J Am Soc Nephrol. 2010;5(7):1261–7.

15. Yi H, Fukagawa M, Yamato H, Kumagai M, Watanabe T, Kurokawa K. Prevention of enhanced parathyroid hormone secretion, synthesis and hyperplasia by mild dietary phosphorus restriction in early chronic renal failure in rats: possible direct role of phosphorus. Nephron. 1995;70(2):242–8.

16. Combe C, Aparicio M. Phosphorus and protein restriction and parathyroid function in chronic renal failure. Kidney Int. 1994;46(5):1381–6.

17. Lopez-Hilker S, Galceran T, Chan YL, Rapp N, Martin KJ, Slatopolsky E. Hypocalcemia may not be essential for the development of secondary hyperparathyroidism in chronic renal failure. J Clin Invest. 1986;78(4):1097–102.

18. Silver J, Naveh-Many T, Mayer H, Schmelzer HJ, Popovtzer MM. Regulation by vitamin D metabolites of parathyroid hormone gene transcription in vivo in the rat. J Clin Invest. 1986;78(5):1296–301.

19. Martin KJ, Gonzalez EA, Gellens M, Hamm LL, Abboud H, Lindberg J. 19-Nor-1-alpha-25-dihydroxyvitamin D2 (Paricalcitol) safely and effec-

tively reduces the levels of intact parathyroid hormone in patients on hemodialysis. J Am Soc Nephrol. 1998;9(8):1427–32.

20. Tan Jr AU, Levine BS, Mazess RB, Kyllo DM, Bishop CW, Knutson JC, et al. Effective suppression of parathyroid hormone by 1 alpha-hydroxy-vitamin D2 in hemodialysis patients with moderate to severe secondary hyperparathyroidism. Kidney Int. 1997;51(1):317–23.

21. Sprague SM, Llach F, Amdahl M, Taccetta C, Batlle D. Paricalcitol versus calcitriol in the treatment of secondary hyperparathyroidism. Kidney Int. 2003;63(4):1483–90.

22. Nemeth EF, Steffey ME, Hammerland LG, Hung BC, Van Wagenen BC, DelMar EG, et al. Calcimimetics with potent and selective activity on the parathyroid calcium receptor. Proc Natl Acad Sci U S A. 1998;95(7): 4040–5.

23. Joy MS, Kshirsagar AV, Franceschini N. Calcimimetics and the treatment of primary and secondary hyperparathyroidism. Ann Pharmacother. 2004;38(11):1871–80.

24. Block GA, Martin KJ, de Francisco AL, Turner SA, Avram MM, Suranyi MG, et al. Cinacalcet for secondary hyperparathyroidism in patients receiving hemodialysis. N Engl J Med. 2004;350(15):1516–25.

25. Lindberg JS, Culleton B, Wong G, Borah MF, Clark RV, Shapiro WB, et al. Cinacalcet HCl, an oral calcimimetic agent for the treatment of secondary hyperparathyroidism in hemodialysis and peritoneal dialysis: a randomized, double-blind, multicenter study. J Am Soc Nephrol. 2005;16(3):800–7.

26. Tominaga Y, Tanaka Y, Sato K, Nagasaka T, Takagi H. Histopathology, pathophysiology, and indications for surgical treatment of renal hyperparathyroidism. Semin Surg Oncol. 1997;13(2):78–86.

27. Aggarwal HK, Jain D, Kaverappa V, Kaushik S, Yadav S. Role of cinacalcet in the treatment of secondary hyperparathyroidism in chronic kidney disease. Russ Open Med J. 2013;2(3).

28. Fukagawa M, Kitaoka M, Yi H, Fukuda N, Matsumoto T, Ogata E, et al. Serial evaluation of parathyroid size by ultrasonography is another useful marker for the long-term prognosis of calcitriol pulse therapy in chronic dialysis patients. Nephron. 1994;68(2):221–8.

29. Kitaoka M, Onoda N, Kitamura H, Koiwa F, Tanaka M, Fukagawa M. Percutaneous calcitriol injection therapy (PCIT) for secondary hyperparathyroidism: multicentre trial. Nephrol Dial Transplant. 2003;18 Suppl 3:iii38–41.

30. Koiwa F, Kakuta T, Tanaka R, Yumita S. Efficacy of percutaneous ethanol injection therapy (PEIT) is related to the number of parathyroid glands in haemodialysis patients with secondary hyperparathyroidism. Nephrol Dial Transplant. 2007;22(2):522–8.

Chapter 11
Vitamin D in Psoriasis

Kevin Man Hin Luk, Vin Tangpricha, and Suephy C. Chen

Case Presentation

A 59-year-old African American male presented to clinic for evaluation of plaque-type psoriasis. The clinical diagnosis was confirmed by biopsy of the right forearm plaque, which revealed prominent parakeratosis with an absent granular cell layer, epidermal acanthosis with suprapapillary plate thinning, and superficial dermal mononuclear perivascular cell infiltrate consistent with psoriasiform dermatitis. The patient was placed on 20 mg acitretin daily, calcipotriol cream daily on weekdays, and clobetasol ointment daily during weekends and experienced symptomatic improvement. At that time, all thick leg plaques were cleared.

K.M.H. Luk (✉) • V. Tangpricha, M.D., Ph.D.
Emory University School of Medicine, Atlanta, GA, USA
e-mail: kluk@emory.edu; vin.tangpricha@emory.edu

S.C. Chen, M.D., M.S.
Emory University Department of Dermatology, 1525 Clifton Road, 1st Floor, Atlanta, GA 30322, USA

© Springer International Publishing Switzerland 2016
V. Tangpricha (ed.), *Vitamin D*,
DOI 10.1007/978-3-319-26176-8_11

However, the patient's triglycerides were found to be elevated at 569 mg/dL in non-fasting conditions and 528 mg/dL in fasting conditions (normal range, 35–160 mg/dL). Acitretin was decreased to 10 mg daily, and the patient was started on gemfibrozil. Triglyceride levels stabilized at 252 mg/dL within the same month, and the patient was advised to maintain 10 mg daily acitretin dose as long as CBC, CMP, and lipid panels remained within normal limits. The patient subsequently reported psoriasis flares while on 10 mg acitretin daily, and the dosage was increased back to 20 mg daily.

Presently, the patient's psoriasis remains fairly well controlled with approximately 5 % of his body surface area (BSA) affected. The patient remains afflicted with persistent plaques on the upper gluteal cleft with well-demarcated erythematous to violaceous thin plaques and overlying scale. Other significant skin findings include small well-demarcated, mildly erythematous plaques on his elbows and lower legs—most pronounced over lateral portion of the legs—bilaterally. In addition, the patient has hyperpigmented, smooth macules and patches on his trunk. Nail pitting is present on fingernails bilaterally. The patient's face and scalp remain unremarkable. The patient reports dry lips relieved by lip balm. The patient denies hair loss, muscle aches, gastrointestinal upset, nausea or vomiting, or other side effects. Review of systems and physical exam are otherwise unremarkable.

Diagnosis/Assessment

Diagnosis of psoriasis is predominantly based on clinical presentation. The disease is characterized as well-demarcated, erythematous plaques with overlying silvery scale. The plaques are typically symmetrically distributed. Commonly affected regions include: the scalp, extensor elbows, knees, umbilicus, and lumbar back. However, the spectrum of disease is broad, and psoriasis lesions can occur anywhere along the skin surface. It can range from limited localized disease to covering a portion of the BSA. These areas may even involve intertriginous areas (inverse psoriasis), the ear canal, palms, soles, or nails [1]. Psoriasis is typically asymptomatic aside from visible plaque development; however, pruritus complaints have been described. Some other commonly associated signs are the Koebner phenomenon and the Auspitz sign. Koebner phenomenon refers to the development of skin lesions at the sites of skin trauma [2]. The Auspitz sign refers to the tendency of psoriatic plaques to pinpoint bleed after scale removal. Although a common additional finding, the Auspitz sign is neither sensitive nor specific for psoriasis [3].

While psoriasis diagnosis is mainly based on clinical findings, skin biopsy of plaque lesions can be done to rule out other conditions. A 4 mm punch biopsy from involved skin is recommended, but mid-dermal shave biopsy is also adequate [4]. Periodic acid-Schiff diastase (PAS-D) stain of a specimen can help discriminate psoriasis from superficial fungal infections [5]. Histologically, psoriasis is characterized by epidermal hyperplasia and abnormal differentiation of epidermal keratinocytes due to a disordered immune response. Furthermore, parakeratosis, neutrophils in stratum corneum and epidermis, thinned or absent granular epidermal cell layer, or thinning of suprapapillary dermal plates are also observed [6].

Shorter keratinocyte cell cycle times and decreased epidermal turnover contribute to the epidermal hyperplasia [7].

Assessment of psoriasis is largely based on the evaluation of plaque distribution and the objective characteristics (erythema, elevation, scaling) of the lesions. The BSA, psoriasis area and severity index (PASI), psoriasis log-based area and severity index (PLASI), and self-administered PASI (SAPASI) are commonly used psoriasis clinical outcome measurement tools. This patient was initially diagnosed with psoriasis based on a combination of clinical assessment and plaque biopsy for confirmation. Psoriasis severity in our patient was also monitored using the BSA. Our patient fluctuated between mild to moderate psoriasis; moderate psoriasis is defined as involvement of 5–10 % of the patient's total BSA [8, 9]. This can be approximated using the complete palmar surface, including the fingers, which is approximately 1 % of the BSA [10]. Additionally, psoriasis is categorized as moderate to severe if it is disabling or if the face, palm, or sole is involved [8, 9].

The Psoriasis Disability Index is a questionnaire to assess the quality of life in psoriasis and can be used to assess the functional impact of disease [11].

Management

The overall aim of treatment in patients with psoriasis is to utilize the various topical and systemic therapies to reduce cutaneous manifestations of the disease. The severity of a patient's psoriasis is used to determine whether topical or systemic treatment is used. Mild to moderate psoriasis or limited psoriasis is well controlled with topical therapies. Moderate to severe psoriasis may require the addition of systemic therapies for adequate control. Patients with greater than 10 % involvement of his or her total BSA usually need systemic therapy for practicality and adequate effectiveness [12]. The patient in this case is being treated with a combination of topical steroids, an oral retinoid, and a topical vitamin D analog. The patient was also instructed to keep his skin well moisturized.

Corticosteroids have long been established as the first-line treatment for psoriasis. Although the exact mechanism is unknown, topical steroids have anti-inflammatory, immunosuppressive, and antiproliferative actions. The efficacy of the topical steroid depends on inherent potency, lesion location, plaque thickness, and compliance [13]. For example, intertriginous areas and the face are typically sufficiently treated with low-potency steroid cream [14, 15]. Potent corticosteroids in solution or foam vehicles are used for afflicted scalp and external ear canal areas or for thick plaques on extensor surfaces [16]. However, topical corticosteroid use can lead to adverse effects such as skin atrophy, lightening, and tachyphylaxis (decreased response after prolonged use). This is especially apparent with long-term use of more potent corticosteroids [17].

Acitretin is a common systemic therapy for psoriasis. Acitretin belongs in the retinoid family and is thought to work by controlling cellular differentiation and proliferation, reducing inflammation and keratinization, and inhibiting neutrophil chemotaxis [18].

As illustrated by our case, one of the most common side effects is hyperlipidemia; 20–40 % of patients on acitretin report elevated triglycerides, while 10–30 % of patients report hypercholesterolemia. The greatest elevation is seen in triglycerides. Patients predisposed to developing hypertriglyceridemia with acitretin use include those with diabetes mellitus, obesity, increased alcohol intake, or a family history of these conditions. Hypercholesterolemia with acitretin use manifests as elevated very low-density lipoprotein (VLDL) and low-density lipoprotein (LDL) fractions with a parallel decrease in the high-density lipoprotein fraction. Thus, acitretin increases the LDL/HDL ratio or atherogenic index, which directly correlates with increased risk of cardiovascular disease. Therefore, fasting lipids should be regularly checked in patients receiving acitretin. Because dyslipidemia is dose-related for acitretin, dietary maintenance and/or acitretin dosage reduction has proven effective in controlling side effects. Gemfibrozil is also recommended, to which our patient responded well [19].

Role of Vitamin D in Management of Psoriasis

Topical vitamin D analogs have recently been shown to best act as either a synergistic adjuvant to topical corticosteroids or as first-line monotherapy itself. Common vitamin D analogs include calcipotriene (calcipotriol), calcitriol, and tacalcitol. When compared to topical corticosteroids, topical vitamin D analog monotherapy has comparable efficacies with a more favorable side effect profile in the treatment of psoriasis. However, the two treatments have been shown to be more effective in combination than either alone [20].

The mechanism of action of vitamin D analogs in psoriasis has not been fully elucidated yet. However, the data suggests an immune-based mechanism. Calcipotriol has been observed to have a substantial effect on epidermal keratinization and proliferation; it also has a more selective effect on CD45RO+ and CD8 T cell subsets. CD45RO+ T cells are memory-effector cells in human skin. CD8+ T cells have been shown to be the predominant T cell subset present in chronic plaque psoriasis, whereas CD4+ T cells are predominant in early psoriatic lesions. These are pathogenically relevant to psoriasis, as apoptosis of these cells leads to psoriatic lesion improvement [1].

There are currently no controlled, clinical trial-based guidelines on how best to use this combination therapy. Patients who receive combination therapy must be monitored for adverse effects. Side effects may include the aforementioned topical steroid adverse effects and skin irritation from topical calcipotriene. The risk of developing hypercalcemia secondary to topical vitamin D treatment is low when applied appropriately [21]. Furthermore, it is known that acidic products may inactivate topical calcipotriene. Because some topical corticosteroids are acidic, it is recommended to advise patients to apply the topical corticosteroid and vitamin D analog at separate times, once daily [22].

Finally, using emollients and moisturizers to soften and hydrate the skin is recommended as an adjunct to psoriasis treatment. This has been shown to reduce pruritus, tenderness, and the potential to undergo Koebnerization [23].

Outcome

The patient remains stable on 20 mg acitretin daily, topical calcipotriene cream applied twice a day on weekdays, and topical clobetasol ointment twice a day on weekends. Recent laboratory work showed an unremarkable CBC. CMP was also unremarkable with a creatinine of 0.9 mg/dL, down from his 2-year baseline of 1.2 mg/dL (normal range, 0.6–1.2 mg/dL). Lipid panel showed an elevated triglyceride of 327 mg/dL, but it is relatively decreased compared to the patient's triglyceride of 644 mg/dL 5 months prior (normal range, 35–160 mg/dL).

The patient was scheduled to follow up with his primary care provider for further medical control of his lipids. In addition, the patient will continue to have his CBC, CMP, and lipids checked every 6 months.

Literature Review

Psoriasis

Global psoriasis prevalence rates vary greatly. Current data suggests that the variation can be seen across age, geographic region, and even distance from the equator. Psoriasis is present in approximately 0.91–8.5 % of adults and 0–2.1 % of children [24]. Various types of psoriasis exist including chronic plaque, guttate, pustular, erythrodermic, and inverse types. Our patient's psoriasis type, chronic plaque psoriasis, is the most common. It accounts for approximately 79 % of adult psoriasis cases [25].

No specific genetic markers have been directly linked with psoriasis. However, psoriasis tends to be concordant among monozygotic twins more commonly than among dizygotic twins [26]. Genetic susceptibility has been connected to various MHC, HLA, and interleukin genes. Among associated genetic loci, PSORS1 on chromosome 6p21 has been deemed a major determinant of psoriasis susceptibility [27, 28]. Other nongenetic risk factors include smoking, obesity, drugs (beta blockers, lithium, antimalarial drugs), TNF inhibitors, vitamin D deficiency, and some infections (HIV or poststreptococcal flares) [29–32].

While the pathophysiology is incompletely understood, it is hypothesized that a systemic autoimmune mechanism in which T lymphocytes, in particular activated memory-effector T cells, and dendritic cells play a central role in the production and activation of inflammatory cytokines. Studies have reported a delay in expression of keratins 1 and 10 (K1 and K10) and overexpression of keratins 6 and 16 (K6 and K16) in psoriatic skin. These are typically seen in normal skin and reactive, healing skin, respectively. Psoriatic erythema and scaling are secondary to hyperproliferation and abnormal differentiation of the epidermis, inflammatory cell infiltration, and vascular changes. The hyperproliferative state of psoriasis is characterized by hyperproliferation of basal cells, shortened keratinocyte cell cycle, and decreased epidermal turnover. Normal keratinocyte cell cycles take approximately 311 h relative to the 36 h in psoriatic keratinocytes. In addition, epidermal turnover in normal skin takes approximately 28 days, while psoriatic skin turns over from the basal to the stratum corneum layer in 4 days time [1].

Vitamin D in Psoriasis Treatment

The major source of vitamin D for the body is the skin. Vitamin D is synthesized in human skin following ultraviolet (UV) light exposure. Approximately 90 % of all vitamin D in the human body is formed in the skin though UV radiation. While vitamin D-fortified milk is an additional source in the American diet, very few natural foods contain sufficient quantities of vitamin D. In addition to helping bones grow, it was recently discovered that vitamin D might play a role in autoimmune conditions of the skin as well [33, 34]. Epidermal keratinocytes are the primary source of vitamin D synthesis but also contain the enzymatic machinery necessary to metabolize vitamin D into its active metabolite 1,25-dihydroxyvitamin D3 [calcitriol or 1,25(OH)2D]. In normal skin physiology, vitamin D contributes to epidermal development from the basal layer to the stratum corneum [1, 35, 36].

Topical vitamin D agents inhibit keratinocyte proliferation, induce keratinocyte differentiation or apoptosis, and modulate activity of immune cells without significant effect on serum calcium homeostasis. It also promotes formation of the permeability barrier and modulates humoral and cellular immune systems and the hair follicle cycle [1]. In fact, keratinocytes express vitamin D receptors (VDRs) and are able to respond to the vitamin D it produces in an autocrine fashion [35].

The physiologically active form of vitamin D, 1,25-dihydroxyvitamin D [1,25(OH)2D], and the VDR have roles in most steps of epidermal development and keratinocyte differentiation. They regulate the synthesis of lipids that are critical to maintain the permeability barrier of the stratum corneum. Vitamin D also regulates the synthesis of loricine and filaggrin in the stratum granulosum. Furthermore, it regulates the synthesis of keratins K1 and K10, involucrin, and transglutaminase in the stratum spinosum. It also modulates cellular proliferation in the stratum basale. Therefore, if the active form of vitamin D is deficient or decreased or VDR function is lost, the basal layer hyperproliferates. This disrupts the differentiation of the epidermis. Because the erythematous scaling plaques in psoriasis are due to keratinocyte hyperproliferation and abnormal differentiation, it is thought that the level of response to vitamin D analog therapy depends on the VDR expression level in keratinocytes. This was seen in mice studies where responsiveness corresponded to VDR levels in lesional skin. Vitamin D analogs' antiproliferative effects and upregulation of VDR expression on epidermal keratinocytes help enhance their regulatory role on cell differentiation and proliferation [1, 34]. Landmark clinical trials have demonstrated excellent efficacy and safety profiles related to vitamin D analog treatment of psoriasis [37].

Another possible mechanism implicates integrin expression. Integrins are altered in psoriatic skin, which results in loss of their adhesive ability and keratinocyte overproliferation. Vitamin D analogs have been shown to normalize integrin distribution, namely, CD 26, ICAM-I, and HLA DR, along the dermal-epidermal junction [38].

Clinical Pearls/Pitfalls

- Psoriasis classically presents as erythematous plaques with overlying silvery scale. The lesions typically present on extensor surfaces and may exhibit the Auspitz sign. The Koebner phenomenon, lesions appear after trauma to the skin, may also be recorded from the history:
- The pathophysiology behind psoriasis remains to be fully elucidated. However, the current data suggests an immunopathologic component that is possibly related to several specific genetic loci, such as PSOR1.
- Topical treatment is first line. Systemic therapies may be introduced depending on severity of the patient's psoriasis.
- Topical vitamin D analogs as monotherapy or in combination with a potent or ultrapotent topical corticosteroid have become the first-line treatment for psoriasis. The combination has been shown to be more effective and safe than monotherapy with either.

References

1. Soleymani T, Hung T, Soung J. The role of vitamin D in psoriasis: a review. Int J Dermatol. 2015;54(4):383–92.
2. Weiss G, Shemer A, Trau H. The Koebner phenomenon: review of the literature. J Eur Acad Dermatol Venereol. 2002;16(3):241–8.
3. Bernhard JD. Auspitz sign is not sensitive or specific for psoriasis. J Am Acad Dermatol. 1990;22(6 Pt 1):1079–81.
4. Raychaudhuri SK, Maverakis E, Raychaudhuri SP. Diagnosis and classification of psoriasis. Autoimmun Rev. 2014;13(4–5):490–5.
5. Grover C, Reddy BS, Uma Chaturvedi K. Diagnosis of nail psoriasis: importance of biopsy and histopathology. Br J Dermatol. 2005; 153(6):1153–8.
6. Schön MP, Boehncke W-H. Psoriasis. N Engl J Med. 2005;352 (18):1899–912.
7. Weinstein GD, McCullough JL, Ross PA. Cell kinetic basis for pathophysiology of psoriasis. J Invest Dermatol. 1985;85(6):579–83.
8. Henseler T, Schmitt-Rau K. A comparison between BSA, PASI, PLASI and SAPASI as measures of disease severity and improvement by therapy in patients with psoriasis. Int J Dermatol. 2008;47(10):1019–23.
9. Langley RG, Ellis CN. Evaluating psoriasis with psoriasis area and severity index, psoriasis global assessment, and lattice system physician's global assessment. J Am Acad Dermatol. 2004;51(4):563–9.
10. Thomas CL, Finlay AY. The 'handprint' approximates to 1% of the total body surface area whereas the 'palm minus the fingers' does not. Br J Dermatol. 2007;157(5):1080–1.
11. Lewis VJ, Finlay AY. Two decades experience of the psoriasis disability index. Dermatology. 2005;210(4):261–8.
12. Murphy G, Reich K. In touch with psoriasis: topical treatments and current guidelines. J Eur Acad Dermatol Venereol. 2011;25(s4):3–8.
13. American Academy of Dermatology Work Group, et al. Guidelines of care for the management of psoriasis and psoriatic arthritis: section 6. Guidelines of care for the treatment of psoriasis and psoriatic arthritis: case-based presentations and evidence-based conclusions. J Am Acad Dermatol. 2011;65(1):137–74.
14. Kalb RE, et al. Treatment of intertriginous psoriasis: from the medical board of the national psoriasis foundation. J Am Acad Dermatol. 2009;60(1):120–4.
15. Koo J, Blum RR, Lebwohl M. A randomized, multicenter study of calcipotriene ointment and clobetasol propionate foam in the sequential treatment of localized plaque-type psoriasis: short- and long-term outcomes. J Am Acad Dermatol. 2006;55(4):637–41.
16. Samarasekera EJ, et al. Topical therapies for the treatment of plaque psoriasis: systematic review and network meta-analyses. Br J Dermatol. 2013;168(5):954–67.

17. Katz HI, et al. Preatrophy: covert sign of thinned skin. J Am Acad Dermatol. 1989;20(5 Pt 1):731–5.

18. Pang ML, Murase JE, Koo J. An updated review of acitretin—a systemic retinoid for the treatment of psoriasis. Expert Opin Drug Metab Toxicol. 2008;4(7):953–64.

19. Ormerod AD, et al. British association of dermatologists guidelines on the efficacy and use of acitretin in dermatology. Br J Dermatol. 2010;162(5):952–63.

20. Vissers W, et al. The effect of the combination of calcipotriol and beta-methasone dipropionate versus both monotherapies on epidermal proliferation, keratinization and T-cell subsets in chronic plaque psoriasis. Exp Dermatol. 2004;13(2):106–12.

21. Bourke JF, Berth-Jones J, Hutchinson PE. Hypercalcaemia with topical calcipotriol. BMJ. 1993;306(6888):1344–5.

22. Patel B, et al. Compatibility of calcipotriene with other topical medications. J Am Acad Dermatol. 1998;38(6 Pt 1):1010–1.

23. Fluhr JW, Cavallotti C, Berardesca E. Emollients, moisturizers, and keratolytic agents in psoriasis. Clin Dermatol. 2008;26(4):380–6.

24. Parisi R, et al. Global epidemiology of psoriasis: a systematic review of incidence and prevalence. J Invest Dermatol. 2013;133(2):377–85.

25. Tollefson MM, et al. Incidence of psoriasis in children: a population-based study. J Am Acad Dermatol. 2010;62(6):979–87.

26. Brandrup F, et al. Psoriasis in monozygotic twins: variations in expression in individuals with identical genetic constitution. Acta Derm Venereol. 1982;62(3):229–36.

27. Mahil SK, Capon F, Barker JN. Genetics of psoriasis. Dermatol Clin. 2015;33(1):1–11.

28. Sagoo GS, et al. Meta-analysis of genome-wide studies of psoriasis susceptibility reveals linkage to chromosomes 6p21 and 4q28-q31 in Caucasian and Chinese Hans population. J Invest Dermatol. 2004;122(6):1401–5.

29. Raychaudhuri SP, Gross J. Psoriasis risk factors: role of lifestyle practices. Cutis. 2000;66(5):348–52.

30. Ahronowitz I, Fox L. Severe drug-induced dermatoses. Semin Cutan Med Surg. 2014;33(1):49–58.

31. Cullen G, et al. Psoriasis associated with anti-tumour necrosis factor therapy in inflammatory bowel disease: a new series and a review of 120 cases from the literature. Aliment Pharmacol Ther. 2011;34(11–12):1318–27.

32. Orgaz-Molina J, et al. Deficiency of serum concentration of 25-hydroxyvitamin D in psoriatic patients: a case-control study. J Am Acad Dermatol. 2012;67(5):931–8.

33. Holick MF. Vitamin D deficiency. N Engl J Med. 2007;357(3):266–81.

34. Lehmann B, Querings K, Reichrath J. Vitamin D and skin: new aspects for dermatology. Exp Dermatol. 2004;13(s4):11–5.

35. Bikle DD. Vitamin D regulated keratinocyte differentiation. J Cell Biochem. 2004;92(3):436–44.

36. Bikle DD. Vitamin D metabolism and function in the skin. Mol Cell Endocrinol. 2011;347(1):80–9.
37. Holick M, Pochi P, Bhawan J. Topically applied and orally-administered 1, 25-dihydroxyvitamin-D3 is a novel, safe, and effective therapy for the treatment of psoriasis-a 3-year experience with histologic analysis. J Invest Dermatol. 1989;92(3):446–446
38. Savoia P, et al. Effects of topical calcipotriol on the expression of adhesion molecules in psoriasis. J Cutan Pathol. 1998;25(2):89–94.

Index

© Springer International Publishing Switzerland 2016   99
V. Tangpricha (ed.), *Vitamin D*,
DOI 10.1007/978-3-319-26176-8

Printed in the United States
By Bookmasters